The Gland Illusion

T0197955

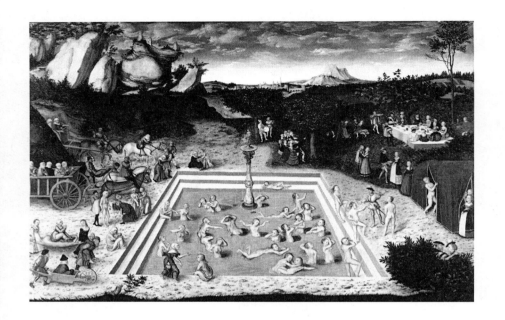

The Gland Illusion

Early Attempts at Rejuvenation through Male Hormone Therapy

JOHN B. NANNINGA, M.D.

McFarland & Company, Inc., Publishers

Jefferson, North Carolina

Frontispiece: The Fountain of Youth, by Lucas Cranach, painted in 1546. The painting shows older, decrepit women being brought to the edge of the pool surrounding the fountain. There they disrobe and enter the pool, where they are transformed into much younger ladies. They exit the pool and enter a tent, where they dress in the latest fashions. They then proceed to a table set with food and drink, then to a dance. The figure atop the fountain is that of Eros, god of love, whom Cranach believed was responsible for regaining youth. (Image courtesy of Art Renewal Center, Port Reading, New Jersey; the original painting is in the Staatliche Museen, Berlin-Dahlem.)

LIBRARY OF CONGRESS CATALOGUING-IN-PUBLICATION DATA

Names: Nanninga, John B., author.
Title: The gland illusion : early attempts at rejuvenation through male hormone therapy / John B. Nanninga, M.D.
Description: Jefferson, North Carolina : McFarland & Company, Inc., [2017] | Includes bibliographical references and index.
Identifiers: LCCN 2016059707 | ISBN 9781476666129 (softcover : acid free paper) ∞
Subjects: LCSH: Organotherapy—History. | Rejuvenation—History. | Hormone therapy.
Classification: LCC RM284 .N36 2017 | DDC 615.3/6—dc23
LC record available at https://lccn.loc.gov/2016059707

BRITISH LIBRARY CATALOGUING DATA ARE AVAILABLE

ISBN (print) 978-1-4766-6612-9
ISBN (ebook) 978-1-4766-2659-8

Front cover: (foreground) Leonardo da Vinci's 1492 drawing of the *Vitruvian Man*; (background) microscopic section of testis tissue sample (iStock)

Printed in the United States of America

McFarland & Company, Inc., Publishers
  Box 611, Jefferson, North Carolina 28640
    www.mcfarlandpub.com

Acknowledgments

I first conceived of writing this book after reading an article in 2002 in *The Pharos*, by Virginia Pruitt, a professor of English at Washburn University in Topeka, Kansas. The subject of the article was Dr. John R. Brinkley, the goat gland surgeon, who practiced in Milford, Kansas. Having grown up in Kansas, I had heard stories about Dr. Brinkley and the goat gland "craze." I sought to learn more about Brinkley and what proved to be a gland era. But it took a few years of gathering information before I had time to sit down and start writing.

Few of the articles, books, and pamphlets were readily available on the medical library shelves. Some were online, but some of the journals were no longer in print and hadn't yet appeared on a Web site. Hence, I made multiple trips to the stacks of the Galter Medical Library at Northwestern University. Several of the librarians there, particularly Ron Sims, special collections librarian, were helpful in digging out information from over a century ago. Also of help were Rumune Kubilius, special projects librarian, and Linda O'Dwyer. Sue Sacharski, archivist at Northwestern Memorial Hospital, aided me in finding information on Dr. Victor Lespinasse.

Different sites in the U.S. and England provided valuable material in composing a meaningful and relatively complete account of my subject. On the West Coast, my first visit was to the Lane Medical Library at the Stanford University Medical Center, where Drew Bourn provided the papers of Dr. Leo Stanley, a Stanford graduate. While reviewing the Stanley papers, I found that Dr. Stanley had left additional papers and memorabilia to the Marin County Free Library, in the Anne T. Kent Room Collection. There Laurie Thompson and Carole Acquaviva provided more material on Dr. Stanley, particularly his tenure as physician at San Quentin Prison. Laurie sent me additional newspaper

Acknowledgments

accounts of Dr. Stanley's obituary. While reviewing various articles by and about Dr. Stanley, I discovered that he had donated additional material to the California Historical Society, in San Francisco. A trip there for a review of Stanley's papers was helped immeasurably by Eileen Keremitsis and Allison Moore. They produced additional articles about Dr. Stanley and the various physicians in the Bay Area with whom Stanley had contact.

The late Dr. James Pick provided a textbook by Serge Voronoff and bibliographies of Drs. Lespinasse and Lydston. He had been a student at Northwestern University Medical School while Dr. Lespinasse was still a faculty member. I have wondered if Dr. Pick intended to write a book similar to mine.

Professor Kevin McKenna, of the Northwestern University Feinberg School of Medicine, provided helpful advice about the subject matter of this book.

The librarians at the Chicago Art Institute were helpful in providing information on Lucas Cranach the Elder.

Genevieve Amaral , graduate student in French and comparative literature at Northwestern University, was helpful in translating correspondence between Alexis Carrel and Serge Voronoff, 1912–13.

I am sure there are some whose names I have omitted, particularly several librarians at the Kansas Historical Library. There was also a helpful librarian at the Junction City (Kansas) Museum Archives, and the volunteer, who kept the library open past closing time so I could finish reading a file on Dr. Brinkley. The librarians at the Wellcome Library, in London, were helpful in providing several books by Serge Voronoff not readily available in the States.

Finally, my son Eric was a great help in guiding me through the word processing program so this book could be completed.

Table of Contents

Table of Contents

Preface

Who doesn't want to live longer, live better? Today, with life expectancy of seventy-six years for men and eighty-one years for women, a person nearing retirement age can look forward to at least a decade of life, hopefully filled with enjoyment and a productive existence. But all too often, these years are marred by illnesses such as cancer, heart disease, and neurological diseases including stroke and various dementias. Prevention of the ill effects of aging currently emphasizes diet, including a reduction of foods containing sugar, weight control, exercise, and remaining mentally active.

Separate attacks on the various illnesses associated with aging have shown some success, but a current trend is to attempt to solve the aging process itself. If we were to do so, the above-mentioned diseases would be reduced in frequency, possibly providing two or three additional decades of reasonably good health.

Science is providing early clues to the aging process. The laboratory of Cynthia Kenyon, at the University of California, has been investigating the life of the lowly roundworm. It has been found that certain genes named daf-2 and daf-16 prolong the life of the worm. These studies have been extended to fruit flies and mice. Humans would be the next logical step in studying the activity of these genes and others influenced by them.

The laboratory of Dr. David Sinclair, at the Paul F. Glenn Laboratories for the Biological Mechanisms of Aging at Harvard, has been investigating "longevity control pathways," searching for agents that will promote these pathways. His research has focused on a group of genes known as sirtuins that are believed to protect against the process of aging. The agent found in red wine, resveratrol, seems to increase the activity of sirtuins.

Preface

A relatively new drug, rapamycin, has been used to prevent rejection in kidney transplants. In testing this drug, first in mice, it was found that mice receiving the drug lived longer than control mice. Rapamycin acts to suppress a protein called TOR, and in doing so, reduces the risk of age-related diseases.

Certain foods with so-called antioxidant effects are thought to reduce cell damage and counteract the aging process. However, some foods with antioxidant properties may not be as healthy as once thought. The idea that oxidation from so-called free radicals is the cause of cellular damage related to aging has been reevaluated by studies indicating free radicals may actually signal a process of cellular repair. Thus, a diet rich in antioxidants may lead to harmful effects in certain individuals. Finally, there are vitamins without which the body could not function properly. In a recent book, *Vitamania,* author Catherine Price lucidly describes the function of all thirteen vitamins, fourteen if choline is included. There is no anti-aging vitamin by itself, but a correct balance will promote good health, and this should reduce the complications of aging that creep into one's well-being. An example is vitamin D, a deficiency of which can lead to osteoporosis and subsequent bone fractures.

All of the above illustrates how science reveals the workings of the human body and points the way to new concepts in providing a longer, disease-free life. But what did our ancestors do to combat the effects of aging? Up through the nineteenth century, aging was considered simply part of life. Some individuals lived into their seventh or eighth decade, or even longer, but these were the exceptions. However, at the turn of the twentieth century, people were living longer and needing to continue working to support themselves and their families, prompting some scientists to experiment with new discoveries such as hormones, which might lengthen the lifespan. This opened a new era of experimentation, some of which was, in retrospect, clearly off-base. Believing in the advances of "modern science," such as the radio, the telephone, and the automobile, a credulous public accepted a variety of practices that today would be called quackery. For many individuals, the lack of scientific knowledge would play a role in supporting certain questionable practices.

This book will focus on an era, sometimes referred to as the "gland era" or an era of "gland therapy," and point out how a certain amount of skepticism should accompany the acceptance of a so-called" new discovery." Certainly, the current investigation of stem cells and gene function should eventually reveal the mystery of aging. There may be false conclusions along the way, but the discoveries in the twenty first century should eventually reduce the costly, debilitating effects of growing older.

Introduction

How lovely is youth
Yet it slips away
If you would be happy, be so
There is no certainty about tomorrow.
—Lorenzo de Medici

The search for eternal youth, or a rejuvenation of the body, has taken many strange routes over the centuries.[1] Ponce de Leon's search for the fountain of youth exemplified the determination to ward off the effects of aging. The consumption of various plant and animal products, including the reproductive glands, has had its day of popularity rejuvenating the aging body. At present, calorie restriction, antioxidants, various fish oils, hormones (including estrogen, testosterone, and growth hormone), stem cells and certain genes, are current areas for research in rejuvenation and longevity.[2] However, rejuvenation and longevity are not synonymous. For example, a baseball pitcher seeking to rejuvenate a failing arm may resort to physical therapy, steroid injections, a special bracelet, snake oil, or surgery. An opera singer may have surgery to remove nodes from her vocal cords in hopes of rejuvenating her singing career. But neither the athlete nor the artist is thinking about living to be one hundred. On the other hand, a person in failing health, for whatever reason, may seek help in rejuvenating his body and, in so doing, add years to his life.

The problem of declining health associated with growing older came into sharp focus during the last two decades of the 19th century.[3] Prior to that, aging was regarded as simply a part of life, and, if a person lived a life of moderation in all things, he or she would conserve a "life force" within the body and delay the aging process. In the eighteenth century, Dr. John Hill's advice to old men for living longer emphasized

4

a "moderate diet" and appropriate exercise. He also warned old men to "avoid foolish fondness for women."[4] But the idea of old age as a disease gradually evolved so that scientists and philosophers at the time began to think of ways to delay aging or to rejuvenate oneself.

During the latter part of the nineteenth century, the concept of a "fixed period" in a man's life rose from the research of Dr. M. Beard, who studied the accomplishments of famous men and came to the conclusion that the productivity of humans reached its peak around the age of forty and then declined.[5] Writers on the history of aging have documented the beginning of age discrimination at this time as employers saw the need to replace older workers, who were described as "touchy" and to some extent resistant to advice and criticism.[6] Evaluation on the job, or for a new position, became based on a youthful physical appearance as a measurement of a man's abilities.[7]

It wasn't just the work of the manual laborer, but the professional life of the "thinking man" that came under scrutiny. In 1892, Dr. William Osler, who would become chief of medicine at the new Johns Hopkins Medical School, addressed the problem of an aging faculty. Osler remarked, "In the fifth and sixth decades, there begins to creep over most of us a change noted physically ... in the silvering of the hair and that lessening of elasticity ... and the change is seen in a weakened receptivity and in an inability to adapt oneself to an altered intellectual environment. It is this loss of mental elasticity which makes men over forty so slow to receive new truths."[8]

Later in his illustrious career, Osler gave his valedictorian address when he was departing from Johns Hopkins to Oxford University.[9] In his speech, he devoted the first part to the need for a university to maintain a certain freshness and the need to be able to change, since "a man of active mind too long attached to one college is apt to breed self-satisfaction, to narrow his outlook, to foster a local spirit and to promote senility. The teacher's life should have three periods, study until twenty-five, investigation until forty, profession [practice] until sixty at which point I would have him retired."[10] To make his point further, Osler borrowed an idea from a novel by Anthony Trollope, *The Fixed Period*, in which an imaginary, self-governing island required everyone over the age of sixty to be euthanized.[11] This would spare the younger citizens of the island the suffering associated with old age and eliminate the need for the government to pay for an unproductive segment of the population. This statement was, of course, a "tongue-in-cheek" remark meant to emphasize Osler's belief that a man's best work was behind him after the age of sixty.

Dr. Harvey Cushing was in the audience and wrote an appraisal of Osler's speech in his biography of Osler: "It required no great degree of intelligence to distinguish between the serious and the jocular in what Osler said, and if rightly read, certainly no one's feelings even if he were past life's median, should have been ruffled in the slightest."[12] But the address did ruffle feelings in some who were in attendance. Newspapers carried stories about Osler's recommending euthanasia ("Oslerization"), and it became necessary for Osler to issue numerous clarifications.[13] One newspaper noted that John D. Rockefeller and Andrew Carnegie would be eligible for extinction.[14] Over the next few weeks, the tempest over Osler's address gradually died down.

Of interest was the fact that Osler spared older women from being retired: "After sixty her influence on her sex may be most helpful, particularly if aided by those charming accessories, a cap and fichu [a three-cornered cape]."[15] Was there a note of condescension in Osler's role for older women or was he expressing the common view of the time?

Osler's address did not calm the fears of an older man employed in an occupation from which he might be dismissed because of old age. Those in occupations requiring hard labor were especially vulnerable. Consequently, what might be the solution to aging? Was it possible to heal and rejuvenate an aging mind and body?

In the eighteenth century, two French anatomists, Joseph Lieutard and Theophile de Bordue, working independently, speculated that blood vessels passing into and from an organ or gland might carry a secretion that played a role in the body's function.[16] In the nineteenth century, the French physiologist Claude Bernard, in studying the function of the liver, introduced the term "internal secretion" to designate the product from a gland or organ.

By the early 20th century, the study of "internal secretions" from various glands led to the realization that these chemical messengers were the key to understanding the functions of the human body. It followed that the use of these glandular secretions could be applied to various health problems in an aging population. The old concepts of the body's being governed by various "humors" or electrical energy gradually became obsolete.

Introduction

This book is about some of the early attempts to harness the discovery of internal secretions (later named hormones) to the idea of rejuvenation. I maintain that the use of gland therapy in that era was not illogical, considering the emerging discoveries of the time. The idea of using the testis or ovary as a transplant for the purpose of rejuvenation might seem bizarre today, but it was not inappropriate, given the state of knowledge then. The ability to measure certain glandular deficiencies would not be developed until later in the twentieth century; hence, there were no objective determinations of measuring the function of a particular gland and correcting the deficiency.

It wasn't just human glands that were used as a source of rejuvenation therapy; monkeys, goats, and sheep were also donors. The fact that foreign material was being inserted or injected into the human body didn't stop various practitioners from using glands or glandular products to turn back the clock in their patients. Perhaps the idea of putting a particular part into a human reflected on the conflation of flesh and machine that evolved in the early 20th century.[17] Quacks rapidly seized the idea of gland therapy and promoted new products that a naïve public accepted without question. And the efforts of orthodox physicians, using products derived from various glands to rejuvenate their aging patients, were greeted with enthusiasm by the public and the press. The story of rejuvenation in this era was not just one of questionable practices and inflated claims, but, as Chandak Sengoopta has pointed out, "The fear of old age and death interacted with the modernist faith in science to open a strange and not necessarily irrational field of research."[18]

Scientists and physicians engaged in rejuvenation and combating the aging process were often those with academic credentials. However, there were those among them who abandoned objectivity in evaluating their results and drifted toward quackery. As a group, the story of these practitioners is one of extending the possibilities of gland therapy to a credulous public eager to regain fleeting youth.

As this era unfolded, it wasn't just rejuvenation that was sought. A variety of mental and physical ailments, some associated with aging, some not, gained the attention of physicians who began to use gland therapy in their practices to treat a variety of complaints. At this time, there were few bona fide pharmacological agents available, and the use of glands was considered a valuable addition to the physician's armamentarium.

Introduction

This book will focus on the use of the testis as a gland of promise in rejuvenation. While the ovary was recognized as the source of female internal secretions, its use as an oral preparation or transplant never achieved the popularity or the notoriety of the testis. Interest in ovarian transplantation or the injection of an ovarian emulsion waned with the discovery of estrogen.[19]

The following chapters describe the attempts of various practitioners to bring the benefits of the sex glands to those seeking a renewal of mind and body. Readers interested in the history of science and medicine should find the accounts of patients, particularly men, seeking to regain lost youth from glands fascinating and at times amusing. In one sense, the use of the testis was the Viagra of the early 20th century. Included is a chapter on quackery, a term the reader may conclude applies to the practices of the physicians described herein. But the word quackery leads to a definition of more than a few sentences. In the late nineteenth and early twentieth centuries, those doctors practicing gland therapy thought they were on the leading edge of medical science. And because the results cited by the doctors and scientists of this era seem, at times, miraculous, there is a chapter on the placebo effect, which accounted for the response in most, if not all, of the recipients of the gland treatments.

Today, an aging population is "likely to be seen as a burden and a drain on resources."[20] Hence, the fear of aging and loss of a job to a younger worker has created a market for products aimed at making the user look and feel years younger. These products are advertised as eliminating the effects of aging such as gray hair, arthritis, baldness, memory loss, wrinkles, sluggish bowels, frequent urination, flabby muscles, depression, loss of libido, and erectile dysfunction (impotence). Some products designed to correct these problems have a proven pharmacological basis, but others of questionable value are marketed as "scientifically documented," or loosely linked to a new discovery and endorsed by "thousands of satisfied users." The ailments of an aging public today are not too different from those a hundred years ago. Then, too, they sought the new discoveries of their era that would aid in restoring youth.

Note that the terms testis and testicle are synonymous. One or the other is used, depending on whether the subject of a particular chapter used one or the other term. The words transplant, graft, and implant are often used synonymously, although transplant usually refers to an organ being placed surgically within the body and attached to the appropriate blood vessels, whereas graft often refers to a body part being placed on the surface, such as a skin graft. Implant usually refers to a material or device inserted into the body, such as a knee or hip prosthesis. One of these terms will be used in a particular chapter, again depending on its use by the particular author.

1

Glands

"In physiology it always depends on the idea that there is a use for everything. Today we still look for the use of these parts." —Claude Bernard, 1857(?)

In 1889, the famous French neurologist and physiologist Charles Édward Brown-Séquard astounded the scientific community by announcing at a meeting in Paris that he had injected himself with an emulsion made from dog and guinea pig testicles for the purpose of rejuvenating himself.[1] Brown-Séquard was seventy-two years old and had suffered fatigue and problems with his bowels, urinary bladder, and lower extremities, all attributable to aging. After several injections of the testicular fluid, he noted a "radical change took place over me and I had ample reason to say and write that I gained all the strength I possessed a good many years ago." He then discontinued the injections for about six weeks and claimed a return of the weakness he experienced before the injections. This simple experiment reinforced his belief that the testicular preparation had produced a beneficial effect that was not simply "autosuggestion" (placebo effect).[2]

The belief in this method of rejuvenation, using the reproductive gland, was based on the observations of cattlemen and farmers that castrating an animal altered its growth and behavior, and pointed to some factor that, in the case of the male animal, maintained its virility. Consequently, Brown-Séquard concluded that the injection of the fluid from the testicle could be a new and exciting pathway to the fountain of youth and relief from the symptoms of aging. Also, in the nineteenth and early twentieth centuries, it was believed that masturbation was a debilitating act; hence, the containment of semen was regarded as a means of maintaining moral and physical strength.[3]

The Gland Illusion

An early attempt to document the presence of a secretion from the testicle, not just the production of sperm, was an experiment by A.A. Berthold, in 1849, at the University of Gottingen.[4] In this experiment, Berthold transplanted the testicles from young roosters into their abdominal cavity. The roosters subsequently displayed the behavior of normal males; that is, "they crowed lustily ... and fought with other roosters and showed the usual reaction to hens." Two castrated roosters behaved as capons. Berthold deduced that there must be a product secreted from the testicle that influenced the appearance and behavior of the roosters. By removing the testicles from their normal site, the effect of nerves to the testicles was obviated. Berthold's experiment did not seem to stimulate much interest in the idea of a secretion from the testicle entering the bloodstream and maintaining the sexual characteristics of the animal. Others were reported to have failed in an attempt to repeat the experiment, and, for the next two decades, the concept would lie dormant.[5]

But prior to Berthold's report, the famous British surgeon and anatomist John Hunter reported transplanting a testicle from a rooster into its "belly" and found the testicle had acquired a blood supply.[6] There are conflicting impressions of Hunter's experiments as to whether a testicle transplanted into a hen altered the hen's "natural disposition." Hunter's experiments suggested he was more interested in transplantation itself than in establishing if there was a factor secreted by the testicle.[7] Thus, to Berthold goes the credit for establishing that a secretion from the testicle enters the bloodstream and affects the animal's virility.

Shortly after Brown-Séquard's report in Paris, an editorial appeared in the *British Medical Journal* titled "The Pentacle of Rejuvenescence," which conveyed the "extraordinary nature" of his presentation.[8] The editorial concluded that Brown-Séquard's statements should be confirmed by other "self-experimenters," before his results were likely to meet acceptance. The use of the term "pentacle" implied there was an element of magic in the results.

The English translation of Brown-Séquard's report appeared in the British journal *Lancet* on July 20, 1889. News of the article spread quickly, for in the United States on August 14, 1889, James Galvin, a pitcher for the Pittsburgh Alleghenys (now Pirates) was injected with an "elixir," as it was termed, made from a testicle (source unknown) before a game with Boston. Galvin was the winning pitcher, in addition to hitting a triple, and, according to the press, "If there still be doubting Thomases who concede no virtue in the elixir, they are respectfully referred to Galvin's record in yesterday's Boston-Pittsburgh game. It is the best proof yet of the discovery."[9] Note there didn't appear to be any attempt to hide this treatment from the press. The *Pittsburgh Commercial Gazette* even published the names of the three physicians who were evaluating the "juice." However, the next day, enthusiasm for the testicular product was tempered by a report that the "elixir of life" fad had evidently completed its term. A couple of reporters had been sickened by the experimental injection of the "stuff."[10] On August 17, the *Commercial Gazette* carried a report from Cincinnati in which the testicular product was now labeled the "Elixir of Death" because of severe illness caused by the injections.[11] A local doctor who supplied the injections warned that the emulsion "spoils quickly." Thus the fad seemed to end relatively quickly. It would be a century before the practice of administering "performance enhancing drugs" to athletes arose again.

Galvin's injection of the "elixir" didn't seem to have any lasting effect, as he gave up ten runs in his next start, although his team won the game by scoring fifteen runs.[12] How many injections Galvin received during the remainder of his career is unknown. He was baseball's first three-hundred-game winner, and, earlier in his career, pitched two seasons in which he won forty games.[13] But by 1892, Galvin was out of baseball. He became an umpire for a short time, then owned a tavern in the Pittsburgh area. He died on March 7, 1902, at the age of only forty-five.

At almost the same time as Galvin was receiving his performance-enhancing injection, an article appeared in the *New York Medical Journal* about the use of a testicular product.[14] The author was Dr. William Hammond, former surgeon general, who served under President Lincoln from 1862 to 1864. In this article, Dr. Hammond reported his experience, using a testicular emulsion from a ram. He chose to treat himself first so he might experience any ill effects from the injection before using it to treat others. Although Dr. Hammond denied any particular infirmity for which he was using the injection, he found the injection relieved pain in his left shoulder, the result from a fall the previous year. Two days later he repeated the injection, but this time pain and swelling occurred at the injection site. The swelling required the incision and drainage of "pus." Apparently satisfied there were no serious effects from the injection, at least nothing worse than the need to drain the injection site, Hammond proceeded to treat nine patients with the testicular fluid. A more cautious physician might have repeated several more injections on himself, using a fresh preparation before proceeding further.

The conditions for which Hammond treated these individuals included cardiac symptoms, rheumatism, lumbago, stroke, impotence, and a woman with "melancholia and fixed delusions."[15] In Hammond's judgment, all except the woman experienced some degree of improvement. One man, age fifty, who suffered from "cardiac weakness" was able to walk four miles after the injection. Two men, ages thirty-four and thirty-six, complained of impotence. After their injections, they noted marked improvement in their condition and a feeling of "mental exhilaration." In a sense, Hammond was using the injections as the Viagra of this era.

Hammond did suspect that there might be an element of "auto-suggestion" in these favorable responses. Therefore, in an attempt to discern whether there could be what today would be called a placebo effect, Hammond gave two injections to a man complaining of lumbago. This man had reported improvement from these injections. Hammond then gave a third injection, but injected water instead. The patient reported that this last injection had done him no good, so Hammond repeated an injection, this time using the testicular emulsion. This time the man reported that he "felt entirely well."[16] It is possible that the injection of water caused minimal discomfort; hence, the patient may have felt the injection wasn't strong enough and might explain his failure to discern any benefit from the injection. Hammond didn't comment if the injections of the testicular emulsion were particularly painful. At any rate, this simple experiment reinforced Hammond's belief in the therapeutic benefit from the testicular emulsion.

Note that Hammond used the testicular product for specific complaints and not as a means of overall rejuvenation or prolonging life. He believed the "juice of the testicle" was a "valuable addition to our material medica."[17] And he downplayed the rejuvenation aspect of the "juice" when he wrote, "It is only the sensational newspapers that speak of it as an 'elixir of life' or as an agent capable of making men young again."[18] Thus, only a few months after the report of the "elixir," which made Brown-Séquard feel young again, this treatment became a new therapeutic wonder, at least in the opinion of Dr. William Hammond.

The *Boston Medical and Surgical Journal* published this appraisal of the injections of testicular emulsions: "The sooner the general public, and especially septuagenarian readers of the latest sensation understand that for the physically used up and the worn out there is no secret of rejuvenation, no elixir of youth.... We hope we may soon hear the last of Brown-Séquard's disgusting advice to old men."[19] This article also pointed out that because of Brown-Séquard's reputation as a scientist, his report to the *Société de Biologie,* in Paris, attracted more attention than it deserved.

The New York correspondent for *Lancet* summed up the testicular emulsion experience in America when he wrote, "The announcement that this distinguished physiologist had discovered a method of renewing the vigor of youth in the aged was ... received with an incredulous smile by the profession."[20] From various parts of the country, there were reports that "the paralyzed walk, the lame throw away their crutches, the deaf hear, and the blind see." The same treatment failed in the hands of others. Infections of the injection sites were reported, and the need to sterilize the emulsion was stressed by some physicians. But one critic of sterilization claimed this would harm the sperm.[21] Obviously, some believed live sperm were the rejuvenating agent.

By 1893, Brown-Séquard was reporting near miraculous results from the testicle injections.[22] Many of the reported successes came from other physicians who had obtained the "elixir" from Brown-Séquard's laboratory and were using it on their patients, so Brown-Séquard had no immediate knowledge of the specific details about each patient receiving the injection. He did report the use of an ovarian extract, but it was his impression it was not as effective a rejuvenating agent in women as the testicular fluid was in men. However, he cited an "American lady physician," who had used an ovarian injectable product on sixty women, with some benefit. But the ovarian treatment for rejuvenation never seemed to attract the attention of the medical community and the press as did the reported rejuvenating effect of the testicle.

Despite Brown-Séquard's own use of his elixir, his health gradually deteriorated. In the last year of his life, he suffered from phlebitis, rheumatism, and finally, a fatal stroke.[23] Could the repeated injections of his testicular emulsion have caused or contributed to these problems? The repeated challenges to his immune system from the foreign matter, which undoubtedly contained cellular elements from the testicle, may have shortened his life. However, there don't appear to be any writings to suggest he came to fear or regret using what he believed to be his rejuvenating discovery.

Brown-Séquard died in 1894, at the age of seventy-seven.[24] His obituaries cited his brilliant research in defining the nerve tracts in the spinal cord. He was also credited with being the first to demonstrate that the removal of the adrenal glands was fatal, thus establishing the fact that a vital secretion was produced by the adrenals. However, his research on rejuvenation, questionable in its conclusions, did point the way to continued research on the concept of internal secretion.[25] It was during this time that an important discovery was made in the field of gland function.

In 1891, Dr. George Murray, a house staff physician at University College in London, encountered a forty-six-year-old woman, who complained of languor and sensitivity to cold.[26] Her relatives noted she had become slow in speech and in performing daily activities. On examination, no thyroid gland was palpable. Dry skin and hair loss were also noted. These findings pointed to a loss of thyroid function. Dr. Murray recalled experiments by Dr. Victor Horsley in which removal of the thyroid ultimately resulted in the death of the research animal. Dr. Murray felt a relatively urgent need to correct the woman's suspected thyroid deficiency. Therefore, he proposed to the patient that a thyroid gland be obtained from a freshly killed sheep and an extract made from the gland. This extract would then be injected into her. The woman "consented promptly" to the trial. After obtaining a thyroid gland, Murray compressed it tightly in sterile muslin and collected the fluid as it oozed from the gland. This fluid was then injected into the patient and, after a series of injections, her overall condition improved dramatically. Some years later, it was found that an oral preparation could be made from thyroid tissue, thus obviating the need for injections. This lady lived to the age of seventy-four, dying from heart failure in 1919.[27] This experiment further substantiated the concept that glands produced vital internal secretions.

Another discovery was made in this era, indicating that glands produced vital internal secretions. In 1893, Dr. George Oliver noted that an extract from the adrenal gland produced a marked rise in blood pressure when injected into the circulation of an animal.[28] Oliver took an extract from an adrenal gland to the laboratory of Dr. Edward Sharpey-Schafer, a physiologist at the University of London. After watching Schafer complete an experiment on a dog, Oliver persuaded him to inject the adrenal extract into the dog's venous system. To Schafer's amazement, the adrenal extract caused a sudden rise in blood pressure. This demonstration was further evidence that a product from a gland produced a physiological response. This adrenal secretion would later be named adrenalin (epinephrine).

In 1905, the physiologist, Ernest Starling, summarized the discoveries involving glands.[29] Previously, Starling and his associate William Bayless had discovered a secretion from the small bowel, which caused the pancreas to produce enzymes necessary for digestion. To name the products from the various glands, Starling coined the term "hormone," derived from the Greek word "to arouse." This term applied to the various secretions produced by the glands of the body. The hormones were carried usually by the bloodstream from the organ or gland in which they were produced to the various structures where they caused an effect. No longer was the nervous system by itself or an ill-defined "life force" the mechanism that sustained life.

There were other developments during this period that facilitated the investigation of hormones. One was the invention of the hypodermic needle, through which a liquid or semi-liquid could be injected into the body, thus facilitating the rapid passage of the injected product into the circulation. Ingesting a pill or capsule composed of a gland might result in the digestion of the glandular material, rendering it inactive. Credit for the initial use of a hollow needle and syringe went to Dr. Alexander Wood, in Edinburgh, Scotland. Wood used his invention to inject the newly discovered drug, morphine, to relieve pain and treat "nerve conditions."[30]

Another important discovery during this period was the development of anesthetic agents, chloroform and ether, which, along with morphine, allowed experiments to be performed on animals without causing the animal to writhe in agony, despite being tied down. This provided a stable operating field in which to perform careful dissection of a particular gland. This advance removed somewhat the objections of antivivisectionists, who opposed live demonstrations before medical students and other interested observers.

These advances, along with the use of carbolic acid as a means of sterilizing surgical instruments, contributed to the safe removal of a gland and reduced the chances of a fatal outcome of the experiment caused by the surgery itself.[31] By removing a particular gland, physiologists could study the results of the absent gland and make a judgment about the function of the gland. For example, the removal of the pancreas resulted in the appearance of sugar in the urine, a condition that became known as diabetes mellitus.[32] Removal of the testicles and the effect on the male animal was discussed earlier.

The discoveries made in the study of glands and internal secretions prompted the creation of extracts made from a variety of body parts. These products were used to treat a variety of illnesses because, in many cases, the exact cause was not known. The term "organotherapy" has been applied to this practice.[33] The testis, ovary, spleen, thyroid, thymus, kidney, pituitary gland, muscle, and parts of the nervous system were sources for these extracts. With the exception of the thyroid, these products were essentially worthless, but their use stimulated further research for true hormones.

In 1917, the first issue of the journal *Endocrinology* was published. In it, one of the editors wrote, "There has been during the recent period, in no department of medicine more activity manifested than that which has characterized the study of the glands of secretion."[34] Indeed, this was an enthusiastic endorsement for an emerging specialty (now termed endocrinology). But the beginning years of the specialty were not without growing pains. Walter Cannon, a highly respected Harvard physiologist, described the early practitioner of endocrinology as "threatened with ridicule and scorn because of wild surmises and fantastic claims of brethren whose imagination outran fact and reason."[35] Another observer of the gland scene described the early days of endocrinology: "The products of the endocrine glands are also particularly adapted to exploitation. When first brought to the attention of the public, there was so much discussion and so much written about them in the press that the demands were made for their therapeutic use long before products which were of value could be discovered."[36]

Obviously, the study of internal secretions and their possible role in rejuvenation tended to veer off course in the early twentieth century.

1. Glands

It wasn't just true discoveries that proved difficult to achieve. Physicians applying the limited findings of scientists in that era to their clinical practice often submitted exaggerated claims of success to medical journals and the press, thus moving therapy in the wrong direction. In retrospect, some of these practitioners would be labeled quacks by today's standards. But in an era when only the clinical impression served as a guide, their enthusiasm carried the day. The efforts of these practitioners were greatly appreciated by those credulous individuals receiving gland therapy, whether for rejuvenation or for a particular ailment, and by the press, who amplified and, at times, exaggerated the results.

2

Dr. Victor Darwin Lespinasse

"We find ourselves embarked on the fog-bound and poorly charted sea of endocrinology."
                                               —Dr. Harvey Cushing

Victor Darwin Lespinasse was born on December 2, 1878, in Aurora, Illinois. As a young man, he became interested in studying medicine and enrolled in the Northwestern University Medical School, graduating in 1901.[1] After interning at Cook County Hospital in Chicago, he became an instructor in urology at Northwestern, a specialty in which he had a particular interest. Among his interests in urology was the function of the testicle and how this gland might be used to treat certain conditions. Lespinasse had read the report by Berthold and others in that era and decided to experiment with transplanting the testicle and studying the results.[2] First he transplanted the testicles of male puppies into the abdominal cavities of three other dogs, similar to what Berthold had performed in roosters. After six weeks, the dogs were euthanized and the abdominal cavities explored. No testicles were found. Next he tried removing the testicles from a group of dogs, slicing the glands to a thickness of 1–2 mm, and placing the slices within the fibers of the muscle of the lower abdomen (rectus abdominis). Six weeks later, the area in which the transplanted slices were placed was biopsied, and he found the slices had "shrunk to one-third to one-quarter of their original size." Therefore, he concluded that the ideal method for transplanting a testicle would be to perform a direct blood-vessel-to-vessel anastomosis to provide adequate blood flow to nourish the gland. However, because of the small size of the testicular artery and vein, he deemed this impossible. Lespinasse had previously developed a technique for joining blood vessels in which magnesium rings were attached to the vessels and then the rings brought together, thus providing an open conduit through which blood would flow. But he didn't believe this technique would work in the relatively small testicular artery and vein. His technique never became popular because of the pioneering effort of Dr. Alexis Carrel, who demonstrated that blood vessels could be joined surgically without any intervening structures.[3] Lespinasse did not document whether any microscopic examination was done on the implanted segments of testicle, which would have established if any blood vessels had grown into the segment of testicle and if there were any apparently viable cells. It is not known how much time elapsed before he attempted to duplicate this questionable experiment in humans, but he would soon have the opportunity.

In January 1911, a thirty-eight-year-old man consulted Dr. Lespinasse about the loss of his testicles. One had been removed during a complicated inguinal hernia repair and the other "lost by accident."[4] The man's chief complaint was that he was "unable to have intercourse." Lespinasse arrived at a solution to the problem rather quickly; that is, he proposed a testicle transplant. He believed this procedure would produce the necessary secretion to correct the problem. The patient agreed to this procedure, and Lespinasse subsequently obtained a volunteer, who agreed to donate a testicle. No mention was made of any payment. Lespinasse commented, "I was surprised at the number of testicles that are available for transplantation purposes."

The operation was performed under anesthesia. The donor testicle was removed and divided longitudinally. The recipient's empty scrotum was opened and a space prepared for part of the gland. Another incision was made in the lower abdomen over the rectus muscle. The muscle fibers were separated and part of the divided testicle was implanted in the muscle; the other half was placed in the scrotum. The incisions were closed and the healing was without incident.

On the fourth postoperative day, the patient experienced a "strong erection accompanied by marked sexual desire." The desire was so strong that he insisted on leaving the hospital to satisfy it. Lespinasse reported that the desire and erectile ability lasted at least two years, up to the time he reported this case at the American Medical Association Meeting, in 1913. Lespinasse waited two years before reporting this procedure in order to evaluate the durability of the transplant. He recognized there may have been a degree of "autosuggestion" resulting from the transplant. Also, the erections may have been triggered by a local reflex caused by the incision and not from any erotic stimulus. This author has observed troublesome erections in patients following surgical procedures to the genitalia. This phenomenon usually resolves after several days.

This case was presented at a local medical meeting in Chicago. Dr. William Belfield, a prominent urologist in Chicago, commented that he was not aware of any literature on testicle transplantation, although he did recall the efforts of Tuffier, in Paris, to transplant ovaries. His impression was that Lespinasse's report "acquires extreme interest."[5]

Apparently, Dr. Belfield was not aware of a report that a testicle transplant had been performed by Drs. Hammond and Sutton in Philadelphia in 1912.[6] These surgeons used the whole testicle rather than dividing it into parts, and the blood vessels were sutured end to end, making it a true transplant rather than simply grafting part of the testicle in the scrotum and the remainder in lower abdominal muscle. Their patient was a nineteen-year-old who had discovered his right testicle had enlarged. Because of progressive enlargement, he sought the opinion of surgeons, who expressed concern that the growth might be cancer and recommended the removal of the testicle. The young man expressed concern about the absence of a testicle in his scrotum after surgery. To allay his concern of a half-empty scrotum, Hammond and Sutton considered placing a sheep's testicle in his scrotum. However, after reconsidering this plan, the surgeons decided to implant a human testicle, when one became available.

The surgery was subsequently scheduled when a testicle became available from an accident victim. The testicle was removed from the victim, flushed with sterile salt solution to remove blood clots, and stored overnight in a solution at 40°F. The next day the patient underwent the removal of the enlarged testicle, which proved to be malignant. The preserved testicle from the accident victim was then sutured in place, attaching the blood vessels as best they could. Today a microscope would facilitate attaching such small vessels. The surgeons observed the newly transplanted gland changed in appearance from a "deathlike syncope to a distinct pink appearance."[7] Except for slight bleeding from the incision, which occurred a week after the procedure, the scrotum healed without a problem. The young man remained in the hospital for twenty-three days, and a month later was examined. To the disappointment of the surgeons, the transplanted testicle had atrophied to the size of a "small knob." However, three months later, examination revealed some increase in the size of the gland. The two surgeons regarded their efforts as "not wholly a failure," because they had demonstrated that the "anastomosis of even these minute vessels is possible, [and that] tissues from subjects dying from injury and free from disease can be removed, preserved, and utilized in living tissues." No mention was made about whether sexual function remained intact, but, with one normal testicle, no impairment would be expected. And no mention was made about whether the young man was satisfied with the cosmetic result.

That same day, Dr. Hammond performed what may have been the first kidney transplant in a human, using a kidney from an accident victim. This victim was likely the same source of the transplanted testicle, making the newly deceased man the first multi-organ donor.[8]

In 1914, Dr. Lespinasse reported a second man in whom he performed a testicle transplant.[9] This man was thirty-eight years old and complained of impotence. After examining him, Lespinasse noted the testicles were "a trifle small and much softer than normal." He concluded the impotence was caused by a lack of internal secretion from the testicles and advised a testicle transplant. No mention was made of trying other remedies, ineffective as they may have been, before resorting to surgery. Subsequently, a donor was found and a testicle transplant performed. The surgery consisted of placing part of the donor testicle in the rectus muscle and, because this patient still had both testicles, the remainder of the gland was attached to one of the recipient's testicles. On the third day after surgery, the patient began to have erections and continued having them daily for a month.

How long the hormone-producing cells of the transplanted testicle would function, if they did at all, remained a question in Lespinasse's mind. As though he had doubts about the effectiveness of transplants, he wrote, "Sexual function is about nine tenths psychic and how much is due to the strong mental stimulus engendered by the operation, and how much is actual functioning Leydig cells [hormone-producing] is impossible to determine."[10] Whatever doubts he had about the transplants did not dissuade him from performing testicle transplants over the next decade. Perhaps the "strong mental stimulus" was the deciding factor.

By 1918, Lespinasse had determined what he believed to be the various causes of impotence.[11] These included castration (by accident or disease), testicular failure or underdevelopment, and "associated internal secretion deficiency." This last term may have referred to thyroid and/or adrenal gland failure affecting the testicle. He believed that removing what he termed "toxic elements," such as smoking and alcohol, would offer some improvement. In addition, he also stressed a proper diet and sufficient exercise, although he didn't offer specific guidelines as to these recommendations. For those individuals who he believed lacked secretions from the testicle, and perhaps from the adrenal glands and pituitary gland as well, he prescribed a "shotgun approach," consisting of capsules or tablets of dried testicle, adrenal glands, and anterior pituitary gland. There were no laboratory tests available in this era to document any specific glandular deficiency. Presumably, an animal source provided the contests of these oral products. Finally, if these measures failed, a testicle transplant was recommended.

In his 1918 publication cited above, Lespinasse described a fifty-five-year-old man, who complained of "diminution of his sexual abilities."[12] Examination of the man's testicles revealed the glands to be reduced in size and "soft and flabby." This individual was thought to be good candidate for a transplant because of the abnormality of the testicles. In preparation for the surgery, Lespinasse remarked that it was always easy to obtain glands for transplantation. The testicles could be obtained from accident victims and suicides. This represents a departure from his previous use of testicles from living donors, presumably because such donors were not as forthcoming, and the report of Hammond and Sutton indicated that glands from the deceased could be used. At any rate, after obtaining a testicle, Lespinasse would immerse the gland in cold physiologic saline or Ringer's solution and place it in an ice chest. He believed the gland could be preserved for twenty-four hours before transplantation, although he presented no evidence to support this statement.

The surgery in this particular patient consisted of dividing the donor testicle into several segments and placing them within the rectus muscle. No mention was made of placing part of it in the scrotum. Possibly, complications had occurred from the scrotal location. Lespinasse wrote that the results of the transplant should be "manifest in a few weeks." He didn't mention the return of erections during the first few days postoperatively, as he did with his first reported patients. And he conceded that, after a few months, the transplant may have been completely absorbed, with the "effacement of any benefits which may have accrued to the patient."[13] Obviously, Lespinasse had become more cautious about interpreting his results.

Note that Lespinasse made no mention of using the testicle surgery to eliminate some of the symptoms of aging such as weakness, fatigue, constipation, loss of libido, and urinary complaints. Rather, he focused on the loss of sexual ability and his attempt to rejuvenate it by supplying the internal secretion from the testicle. Longevity was not his primary goal.

This author made an attempt to determine approximately how many of Lespinasse's patients underwent a second transplant, assuming the first resulted in failure. If certain names reappeared on the hospital's surgical schedule, it was very likely that the previous transplant had failed. While some of Lespinasse's cases were in the surgical logs, the records from 1918 on through the 1920s were missing, despite efforts by the hospital archivist to locate them. Hence, it was impossible to document what the failure rate of the testicle transplant experience might have been.

In 1922, Dr. Lespinasse's name appeared in the press as having admitted to the hospital the son of a wealthy Chicago industrialist.[14] Dr. Lespinasse was referred to as a specialist in gland transplantation. This designation gave a strong hint as to why Harold McCormick, age fifty, was admitted. Mr. McCormick was pursuing an opera singer, Ganna Walska, and he must have felt he needed some special form of rejuvenation.[15] His wife, the former Edith Rockefeller, had departed for Switzerland to study with Dr. Carl Jung, a noted psychiatrist. At some point, Mr. McCormick decided to marry Miss Walska, who had a habit of marrying wealthy men, then shedding them. Dr. Lespinasse was supposed to perform an operation, which would rejuvenate Mr. McCormick by supplying the needed boost to his relationship with Miss Walska.

When Mr. McCormick was admitted to the hospital, the press was on top of the story from the beginning.[16] Word of the admission was leaked to a reporter, who in turn notified his fellow newsmen. They visited the hospital and managed to obtain a list of patients, which included the name of Harold McCormick and his physician, Dr. Victor Lespinasse. The reporters then hastened to Dr. Lespinasse's home, arriving around 2 a.m. After failing to arouse the doctor by ringing the doorbell, they proceeded to throw pebbles at various windows until the doctor opened a window and shouted, "What do you want?" After answering some questions, none too revealing about Mr. McCormick's condition, the doctor slammed down the window. He then called the hospital to warn Mr. McCormick about the intrusive press. But a reporter had tapped Dr. Lespinasse's phone and overheard the conversation between doctor and patient.[17]

The exact details of the surgery were not spelled out in the press, but Mr. McCormick's postoperative course was documented in subsequent accounts. "McCormick out in short time," proclaimed the *Chicago Tribune*.[18] The article went on to say the Chairman of the Board of International Harvester "underwent an operation calculated to restore fading tissues." A hospital spokesperson, wishing to show Mr. McCormick was being treated as an ordinary patient, added that his room cost was $8.00 a day, a "plain room," and the room number was 206. So much for privacy!

A visitor to Chicago, Dr. Royal Copeland, who was health commissioner of New York City, read the paper and commented, "The idea that transplantation was of benefit to Mr. McCormick was pure bunk." Dr. Copeland added, "No man has yet been able to transplant an organ from one animal to another and have it function."[19] No doubt, Dr. Lespinasse would have been highly irritated by Dr. Copeland's critical remark about his practice, assuming he read the article.

Two days later, on June 20, the *Tribune* announced, "Harold McCormick was reported to be traveling back towards youth and renewed vigor at such a swift pace that his attending surgeon, Dr. Victor Lespinasse, abandoned his visit to the hospital."[20] This was based on a statement by Dr. Lespinasse that he would not visit the patient again until the following morning, implying that healing was on schedule and there were no foreseeable complications. The article added that because of the publicity, the doctor was "swamped with appeals from others seeking transplantation operations. He is said to have performed at least half a dozen in the past week, including one yesterday morning upon an aged Illinois Central [locomotive] engineer, who used to drive the Panama Limited." Obviously, Dr. Copeland's criticism went unheeded.

On June 24, Lespinasse clouded the issue concerning the source of testicle used in McCormick's surgery when he issued the statement that no human glands were used.[21] He stated, "The story that any part of any other human body has been or will be used in the treatment of Mr. McCormick has not the slightest foundation in fact." Perhaps this statement was meant to throw off any inquiries as to who might be the donor. But a possible donor of the testicle was rumored to be a young blacksmith. This rumor was bolstered by a bit of doggerel making the rounds in Chicago's society drawing rooms:

> Under the spreading chestnut tree,
> The village smithy stands;
> The smith a gloomy man is he;
> McCormick has his glands.[22]

The *Tribune* did quote a fee of $50,000 for the treatment, which Dr. Lespinasse did not deny. Not surprisingly, on June 29, the *Tribune* announced that McCormick intended to sue the newspapers covering this story for libel, telephone tapping, invasion of sick room, and trespassing on his property.[23] It is not clear what became of this threat.

Mr. McCormick and the diva were married in Paris later that year.[24] On the day of the wedding, he called for her in the house given to her by a former husband and drove to the mayor's office in a limousine, which had been a gift from another husband. The marriage lasted until 1931, when the couple separated. The divorce was said to cost Mr. McCormick six million dollars. He then moved to California, where he took up whistling as a hobby and became skilled enough to give a recital over the radio.[25] Harold McCormick died in California, at the age of sixty-nine, nineteen years after the rejuvenating operation. Perhaps the testicle transplant, assuming that is what was performed, did in some way have a beneficial effect on his life, but it proved to be an expensive procedure.

How long Dr. Lespinasse continued to perform the testicle operations is difficult to determine. He was quoted in *Time* magazine in 1925 as protesting the publicity he had received from the gland surgery. "I have a stack of letters here ... as high as your head from men who want to sell their glands. Some of the prices are very reasonable, too.... There are not many buyers. When the gland operations become more popular, naturally the market will stabilize."[26] Lespinasse did not appraise the market correctly, for there were others performing testicle transplants, as will be described in subsequent chapters.

Dr. Lespinasse's interests were not confined to testicle transplants. Throughout his career, he investigated infertility in the male. He published a paper on the surgical correction of obstruction in the vas deferens, preventing the outflow of sperm, and the blockage that occurs at the junction for the vas deferens and the epididymis.[27] Another contribution to urology was one in which he described abnormalities in sperm, including insufficient numbers, abnormal forms, and reduced motility.[28] These were factors which were just emerging as reasons for male infertility. Lespinasse also utilized direct uterine insemination of sperm in cases in which the amount or quality of sperm were less likely to produce a pregnancy.[29] His knowledge of male infertility was recognized by his peers when he was selected as a discussant of a series of papers on the subject at the 1936 meeting of the American Medical Association.[30]

A relative obscure innovation by Dr. Lespinasse has been recognized by the specialty of neurosurgery. In 1910, he performed the insertion of a cystoscope, an instrument used to view the inside of the urinary bladder, into the choroid plexus of an infant with hydrocephalus for the purpose of cauterizing abnormal blood vessels.[31] This procedure was a forerunner of ventriculoscopy, a procedure used today by neurosurgeons.[32]

In 1946, Dr. Lespinasse was a discussant of a paper on the male climacteric, a term thought to be comparable to the female menopause.[33] In his discussion, he pointed out that older men seek his advice because of impotence, and that testosterone, available in an injectable form, worked occasionally to relieve the problem. No mention was made of a testicle transplant, which he had abandoned some years earlier.

Later that year, Dr. Lespinasse, at the age of sixty-eight, suffered a fatal heart attack. His obituary in the *Journal of the American Medical Association* cited the awards given to him by that organization for his research in infertility.[34] His colleagues at Northwestern remembered him for his "active imagination, friendly and sincere attitude, and his efforts to promote blood transfusions in Chicago Hospitals."[35] The obituary in the *New York Times* did cite his "gland surgery," along with accomplishments in vascular surgery and sterility (infertility).[36]

2. Dr. Victor Darwin Lespinasse

In 2008, in a presentation at the History of Urology Forum at American Urological Association annual meeting, the presenters reviewed the accomplishments of Dr. Lespinasse and concluded he was a "visionary, pioneer, and real founding father of modern clinical andrology."[37] Also mentioned was the fact that Lespinasse "later recognized the clinical shortcomings" of the testicle transplant venture.

On a poignant note, in December 1947, Dr. Lespinasse's widow made a request for a grave marker to the Chicago Wesley Hospital, where her husband had been on the staff for nearly forty years. No reason was recorded, but she was probably short of funds for a memorial. At a meeting of the hospital executive committee, the motion was made and seconded for the purchase of a tombstone. The vote was unanimous in favor of the expenditure. One member commented, "This is a very nice thing to do; it is much better than buying liquor for the interns' party."[38]

3

Dr. George Frank Lydston, Jr.

"But to be a man of genius it is not sufficient to have an idea and push it to the extreme.... Nevertheless, exaggeration is usual, and it is made necessary by minds that must be struck hard."

—Claude Bernard, 1857(?)

George Frank Lydston, Jr., was born in 1858 in a robust, sometimes violent California mining town along the Tuolumne River.[1] The Lydston family had come from Maine, hoping to cash in on the gold discovery. Although somewhat successful, Lydston, Sr., decided to move the family back to Maine because of diminishing returns from the gold fields, plus a series of flash floods that nearly destroyed their home. The financial success in Maine was not what the family expected and they moved again, this time to Chicago. There Mr. Lydston engaged in a variety of businesses, eventually becoming a member of the Board of Trade.

Young Frank Lydston completed his secondary education in Chicago and decided to pursue a career in medicine. His decision was partly influenced by his exposure to local doctors back in California, one of whom he remembered as a "best friend and wisest counselor."[2] Lydston's medical education began at Rush Medical College in Chicago, but after a year, he transferred to Bellevue Hospital Medical School in New York City. There he obtained his medical degree in 1879. Subsequently, he served an internship and surgical residency at several hospitals in New York City before deciding to return to Chicago.[3] He became a faculty member at what was then the Chicago College of Medicine and Surgery, later to become the University of Illinois School of Medicine in Chicago. In 1882, the college appointed him lecturer in genitourinary surgery and venereal disease. During the next two decades, he published numerous articles on a variety of urologic subjects. By 1889, he had acquired enough clinical experience to publish a book, *The Surgical Diseases of the Genitourinary Tract.*[4]

The reports of testicle transplantation (Lydston preferred the term implantation) by fellow Chicagoan Dr. Victor Lespinasse, and by Hammond and Sutton, did not go unnoticed by Lydston, nor did the experience reported by Brown-Séquard. Reflecting on Brown-Séquard's self-injections of testicular fluid, Lydston wrote, "Ever since the publication of Brown-Séquard's experiments—then regarded as fantastic—I had entertained more than a suspicion that the venerable Frenchman was not as foolish as some believed. The formation of the internal secretion theory and comparatively recent establishment of their relations to the welfare of the human body convinced me that there was a germ of truth to Séquard's observations."[5]

At this point in Lydston's career, he was fifty-six years old and decided this was the time to proceed with the implantation of the reproductive glands because of what he believed to be their importance to the other glands in the body and their power to rejuvenate the aging body. Believing it was unethical to subject anyone to "whatever dangers the experiment might involve ... I resolved to perform the experiment on myself."[6] Rather than have a colleague perform the surgery, Lydston decided to implant the gland in himself. He acquired a testicle from a suicide victim and placed it in a jar of salt solution on the windowsill in his office. The temperature on this day, January 15, 1914, hovered around 30°F, cold enough to preserve the gland. The next day, Lydston performed the implant.[7] Local anesthesia consisted of 10 percent Novocain, 1 percent urea, and quinine hydrochloride. Assisting with the procedure was an associate, Dr. Carl Michel.

The procedure consisted of making an incision in the scrotum and exposing the testicle and spermatic cord, onto which the donor testicle, stripped of its outer covering (tunica vaginalis), was sutured. The incision was then closed. The implant was performed in Lydston's office under conditions "as satisfactory as were possible under the circumstances." Imagine the commotion this operation would have caused if Lydston had chosen to perform it in a hospital operating room, where other surgeons and the nursing staff would have become aware of what he was performing and voiced their opinion about this seemingly outlandish self-experiment.

During the next twenty-four hours, Lydston experienced a "marked exhilaration and buoyancy of spirits."[8] This feeling decreased over the next few days because of what Lydston believed to be an "inflammatory exudate surrounding the implanted tissue." On the eighth day after the implant, Lydston felt considerable pain in his scrotum and noticed a small amount of tissue protruding from the incision. He summoned Dr. Michel and the two decided the experiment was a failure and the testicle should be removed. Dr. Michel attempted to remove the testicle, but only about half the gland came out. Consequently, the remaining testicle was left in place. Drainage from the incision continued for about five weeks before healing was complete. Lydston didn't reveal how he coped with this drainage. Six weeks later, the remainder of the testicle was felt to be the size of a "hazel nut."[9]

With his new partial gland, Lydston noted the ability to get by with less sleep. He also observed a drop in his blood pressure and the disappearance of what he termed "cardiac irritability," which he had experienced periodically prior to the implant. In regard to sexual function, Lydston was somewhat vague when he described "what might be expected from the local irritation in any normal [man] at this time of life." This statement suggests that reflex erections might have occurred, and he added that the "psychic effect of the reflex stimulation ... could be markedly beneficial."[10] At least, the patient would believe the implant was successful.

Lydston submitted for publication his experience with the testicular implant and informed a surgeon in New York, Robert Tuttle Morris, that he might want to submit his own case of testicle transplantation for publication. Apparently, Lydston had become aware of Morris's interest in the subject. This prompted Morris to report the case of a man who had suffered a severe injury to both his testicles. This patient had been referred to Dr. Morris by "W.J.M." of Rochester, Minnesota.[11] The surgery on this patient consisted of obtaining a gland from an elderly man undergoing an inguinal hernia repair and dividing it into three segments, one being implanted in the scrotum and the others in the lower abdominal muscles. In the follow-up period, the patient communicated to Dr. Morris that life had become "one blissful day." Later he wrote that he had the opportunity to "exercise the function resulting from the operation [and] the sexual congress was quite normal indeed."

Of note was the fact that Dr. Morris had performed an appendectomy on Lydston in 1889.[12]

Inspired by his new "buoyancy of spirits," Lydston embarked on a series of testicle implants over an eight-year period. Lydston's indications for the operation were senility, male climacteric, hypertension, arteriosclerosis, defective and abnormal psychic sexual development (including homosexuality), dementia praecox (schizophrenia), and loss of testicles (usually by accident).[13] On occasion, Lydston performed an ovarian implant, but his results were not as encouraging as was his experience with the testicle. As an example, Lydston implanted an ovary in a fifty-nine-year-old woman suffering what Lydston described as "nerve wreckage," following pelvic surgery. The woman's ovaries had been removed with the resulting loss of estrogen and the onset of menopausal symptoms.[14] To correct the problem, Lydston implanted an ovary obtained from a sixteen-year-old girl, who died from a skull fracture. The ovary was placed in the left labium majora so it could be palpated relatively easily and removed, if complications occurred. Following the implant, the lady sensed a "marked exhilaration" for a few days. Her "hot flashes" disappeared and she found she needed less sleep than before the implant. Several weeks later, she reported the disappearance of "joint stiffness" and increased physical endurance. Five months later, Lydston examined the lady and could still palpate the ovary. He believed her health would continue to improve, but a year after the implant, she suffered what Lydston described as a "severe nervous shock," and her condition was "very unsatisfactory."[15]

Lydston also reported two young women, who suffered from dementia praecox. In one, an ovarian implant was placed just above the right hip. This lady showed no improvement from the implant. The other young woman underwent an ovarian implant in the right labium majora. This ovary had been refrigerated for a week before implantation. It is inconceivable that there were any viable cells in this ovary. And not surprisingly, an infection developed in the implant requiring drainage. However, the ovary was left in place. Several months later, the patient's mental condition was thought to have improved. This patient reinforced Lydston's belief that dementia praecox was a condition in which "the secretions of the genital glands are greatly perverted."[16]

Hence, Lydston's belief that placing a new ovary in a patient suffering from dementia praecox would establish a normal hormonal milieu. The fact that the ovary could be a week old didn't seem to bother him.

Lydston also implanted a testicle into a sixty-year-old woman suffering from senile dementia. He was interested in whether a sex gland could be transplanted from one sex to the other.[17] This was before the discovery of estrogen and testosterone, and Lydston thought there might be a common secretion from each gland. For example, the secretion from the thyroid is the same for both men and women. The testicle that Lydston implanted in this woman had come from a thirty-year-old man, who died from touching a "live wire." The gland had been refrigerated for four days before being implanted. Four months later the testicle was removed because it had become a source of "disquiet." Lydston did not mention whether the woman was told she was having a testicle implanted inside her; she may have been so mentally impaired that she would not have understood the nature of the surgery. The use of sex glands reflects the difficulty in treating mental disease in this era.

Even though Lydston had limited experience in sex gland implantation, nevertheless he concluded that the concept of implanting the glands to cure a variety of illness and promote rejuvenation offered the key to the arrest of aging. To quote Lydston: "If we ever succeed in impeding the wheels of time in their remorseless grind on human life— and I confess optimism—it is most likely through internal secretion therapy via gland transplantation. The sex gland secretion seems to be the most important secretion as far as its possible effect on increasing efficiency and longevity are concerned."[18] Thus, Lydston concluded that gland implants would serve as a specific treatment for a variety of ailments and because of the rejuvenating effects, the "remorseless grind on human life" would be slowed.

In addition to the gland surgery, Lydston experimented with the injection of emulsions made from various glands and organs.[19] This was similar to the practice of Brown-Séquard and his "testicular emulsion," and to that of Dr. William Hammond referred to earlier, who experimented with an emulsion from a ram's testicle. Lydston recognized the ease of performing an injection rather than surgically implanting a gland. The effect from an injection should, theoretically, produce an effect sooner than implanting an ovary or testicle and waiting for the gland to acquire a blood supply and begin to function.

3. Dr. George Frank Lydston, Jr.

Lydston treated twenty-three individuals with injections from various organs, glands, and other structures. At first he injected guinea pigs with human kidney emulsion to determine if there were any adverse effects from the injection. Then, after observing no ill effects, he injected himself and experienced no adverse effect. Convinced the kidney emulsion was safe, he gave a sample of the emulsion to a colleague to use on a patient with kidney disease. The emulsion proved to be harmless and ineffective in altering the course of the kidney ailment.

Next, Lydston obtained a brain from an accident victim. The brain had been carefully cleaned so that an emulsion made from it was relatively free from contaminants.[20] This emulsion was tested on guinea pigs, and when no ill effects were noted, he injected himself. After several injections, he noted only a "little redness" over the injection sites. Having determined the relative safety of the brain emulsion and noticing no adverse effect on his cerebral function, he injected the emulsion into a trusting, seventy-year-old "medical friend," who was suffering from "neurasthenia." The friend's condition was reported to have improved, but Lydston did not provide any details about the improvement.

Continuing with the brain experiments, this time using the cerebellum, Lydston injected the emulsion into a "healthy volunteer," without testing it on a guinea pig or himself. After the first injection, the volunteer reported that he experienced an "erection and nocturnal emission of semen."[21] On hearing about this response, Lydston must have thought he had found an answer to his male patients' sexual difficulties. However, this volunteer did not experience this phenomenon with further injections. But others who did receive the cerebellar emulsion reported feeling "invigorated." No further mention was made of a specific effect on sexual function. Lydston did make the point that the source of the injection, the brain, was not revealed to these research subjects. He probably wished to avoid any placebo effect which might be associated with a particular gland or organ. Thus, the individuals receiving the injections were more than likely not aware of any risks associated with brain tissue and the possibility of transmitting a disease such as syphilis.

In a final series of patients, Lydston used an emulsion made from a ram's testicle.[22] This practice recalls Dr. William Hammond's self-injection of an emulsion from a ram's testicle. Lydston did not mention Hammond's experience and may not have been aware of it. At any rate, Lydston wanted to evaluate the use of a non-human source. Would it produce a severe reaction, in addition to its possible rejuvenating effect? Lydston tested the emulsion from the ram's testicle on a guinea pig, and when there was no evidence of an allergic reaction, he then injected himself in his thigh. After six doses, he noted only slight swelling and tenderness at the injection sites. His thighs must have been somewhat tender after the multiple injections of the various products. Lydston did not describe the "buoyant feeling" as he had after implanting the human testicle in himself the previous year. Despite this lack of effect, and having determined the emulsion was safe, he proceeded to inject ten men described as "pseudo-impotents and sexual neurasthenics." His diagnoses implied he did not believe these men were completely impotent, but were experiencing "functional" sexual problems. Following the injections, the men reported their condition (presumably impotence) was improved, along with their appetite.[23]

Lydston acknowledged the results from these injections may have been "psychic," although none of the subjects knew a ram's testicle had been the source of the injection material. Perhaps the use of an injection rather than a pill enhanced the anticipated beneficial effect. The response to an injection rather than a pill will be discussed in a later chapter on the placebo effect. When the injection was ineffective, Lydston believed the addition of a preservative may have blunted the action. However, he believed the use of a preservative was necessary as a "partial insurance against carelessness in manufacture and administration." Recall that two sportswriters who received injections of a glandular product the day after the pitcher James Galvin was injected became violently ill. Lydston may have continued to use the testicle emulsions in his practice because the injections were simpler than performing an implant.[24] Yet he continued to perform the implant in selected cases.

If Lydston detected a definite abnormality in the testes of a patient seeking his care, he was more likely to proceed with a testicle implantation. An example was that of a twenty-nine-year-old man who had suffered trauma to one testicle in a football game, and several years later experienced a sharp pain in the other testicle, which gradually shrank in size over several months.[25] The end result was that the man became impotent and lacked "efficiency" in his work. Lydston's examination of the man revealed markedly atrophied testicles. Lydston's solution was to recommend implanting new testicles. The surgery was scheduled when Lydston obtained the glands from a fourteen-year-old boy killed in an accident. Lydston had placed the glands on ice for about thirty-nine hours before surgery. Several days after the implant, Lydston performed a circumcision on the patient because, in Lydston's estimation, the man's foreskin was too long. On the eighth day post-implantation, the man began having "vigorous and painful erections, requiring an ice bag for relief."[26] About three weeks after discharge, the patient reported he was having successful sexual relations. Several months later, Lydston examined the man and found the implanted testicles had atrophied only moderately, and the man had noted an increase in "mental and physical fitness for business." Lydston had this patient examined by Dr. William Belfield, a prominent urologist in Chicago and founder of the Chicago Urological Society, who remarked, "The testicles, while small, are as well developed and apparently normal as in many perfectly virile men who come under our observation."[27]

Lydston was quite pleased with the results in this man when he wrote, "This much is evident, namely, that my implantation work has passed the experimental stage. It would require a degree of skepticism which I am free to say does not inspire me ... to attribute to psychic impress such results as have been obtained."[28] In other words, he dismissed the placebo effect in his results.

In his book, published in 1917, titled *Impotence and Sterility, with Aberrations of the Sexual Function and Gland Implantation*, Lydston summarized his approach to treating impotence.[29] This approach included, first, having a man abstain from "all sources of sexual stimulation." This allowed the sexual desire to build up. A change of scene was also advised, along with avoidance of associations that "excite the passions." Cold showers or sitz baths alternating with hot water were recommended. Nutrition was important. Lydston recommended the diet include malt, cod liver oil, rich milk and cream, meat cooked rare, and alcoholic beverages such as claret, port sherry, or Dublin Stout. Today we know that, if a man's erectile dysfunction is related to poor blood flow and arteriosclerosis, the rich milk and cream would likely exacerbate the problem.

If the above measures were unsuccessful, Lydston recommended a variety of medications including strychnine (used as a central nervous system stimulant), iron tablets, opium, bromide, ergot, digitalis, cantharides (Spanish fly), and pilocarpine. These could be used singly or in combination. Lydston warned of mail-order medications advertised by quacks, and acknowledged the reputation of quacks was based on the influence of the product on the mind of the user. He observed, "An individual who is impotent because of a lack of confidence in his virility is likely to be relieved by ... milk sugar, provided he has confidence in the efficacy of the placebo."[30] Lydston obviously recognized the effect of the placebo.

Lydston's book also recommended another form of therapy for impotence; this was electricity.[31] This treatment included a "faradic bath," the current being applied directly to the spine, perineum, penis, and testicles. Lydston remarked, "The stimulating effect of the static electricity upon the nervous system often is remarkable; some patients say it acts like a 'glass of champagne.'" Another site for electrical stimulation was the prostate. Here the electrode (negative) was passed through the urethra to the level of the prostate, and the positive pole was applied to the spine, thighs, or genitals. An alternative approach was to suspend the penis and testicles in a container of warm water (negative) and hold the positive pole in the patient's hand. No time limit was given, but if the above techniques failed to improve the erectile function, Lydston would recommend a testicle implant.

At this point in his career, some doubt seemed to have blunted his enthusiasm for the testicle surgery when he wrote, "Since the original experiment [on himself], it has become evident that, in most cases, complete atrophy occurs, the time at which it occurs being variable, but in all cases being delayed sufficiently to secure the benefit of the sex hormone for a prolonged period."[32] How long the effect would last was never documented, but Lydston may have thought the effect would be for years, even though the atrophic gland had ceased to function. For that matter, how long would the placebo effect last?

However, there were two instances where Lydston indicated at least some enthusiasm for testicle implantation. One day, when Lydston was entering the elevator in his office building, he met a colleague, Dr. Max Thorek, who remarked to Lydston that a surgeon in Paris, Dr. Serge Voronoff, was transplanting monkey testicles in aging men.[33] Lydston responded by asking Dr. Thorek if he had a minute, to which

3. Dr. George Frank Lydston, Jr.

Thorek replied he always had time for Frank Lydston. The two entered Lydston's office and Lydston motioned Thorek to follow him into an examining room, where Lydston disrobed. Thorek felt a bit uncomfortable until Lydston called his attention to the extra testicle in his scrotum. This was followed by a lecture on the new field of sex gland implantation.

Another episode indicating Lydston's interest in gland surgery involved Lydston and Dr. Morris Fishbein, who would later become editor of the *Journal of the American Medical Association*. In conversation with Dr. Fishbein, Lydston brought up the subject of gland transplantation, and, after a brief discussion, Lydston unbuttoned his shirt, revealing several lumps. When Dr. Fishbein asked about the source of the swellings, Lydston replied, "They are testicles."[34] Lydston must have felt the need to provide an extra boost to his body from the testicles. Fishbein's summation of Lydston was that he was a "remarkable and eccentric man."

Lydston presented his experience with testicle implantation to the Chicago Urological Society on November 15, 1917.[35] Unfortunately, the minutes of the meeting did not include a copy of Lydston's report nor any discussion of the cases. No doubt, the discussion of his paper was lively. Most likely, Drs. Belfield and Lespinasse would have been present and participated in the critique. Curiously, Lydston did not become a member of that organization until 1919, despite having been in practice in Chicago for nearly forty years. There may have been something controversial about his practice, his book, or his medical politics, which led to the delay in the membership's accepting him.

In 1918, Lydston wrote a paper in which he described a sixteen-year-old boy who, as a child, developed orchitis following a vaccination.[36] The boy had not yet matured sexually. Lydston evaluated the lad and determined that a testicle implant would hasten the boy's development. A testicle became available from a victim of carbon monoxide poisoning. The gland was refrigerated for about thirty-two hours before implantation. Sixteen months later, the young man had gained weight, assumed a masculine appearance, and experienced frequent erections. Based on these developments, Lydston concluded his report by stating, "I am convinced my method of sex gland implantation long since has been taken from the purely experimental field, and it now stands on firm ground as a valuable therapeutic resource."[37] It did not seem to occur to Lydston that this boy may simply have been a late-maturing individual and the testicle implant was irrelevant. This was not the first time that hubris emerged from Lydston's implant experience.

Near the end of his career, Lydston reported a case which resulted in an astounding result. A thirty-four-year-old individual consulted him about his beardless condition, scanty pubic hair, and "markedly falsetto voice."[38] This person had never engaged in any sexual activity. His genitalia were described as those of a "one year old." Lydston didn't describe whether the boy/man was short or tall and whether any testicles could be palpated in the underdeveloped scrotum. The abnormalities led Lydston to diagnose "hypopituitarism." Lydston was reluctant to consider a testicle implant for this individual, but at the insistence of the man and his family, he decided to proceed with the surgery. He believed the implanted testicle would supply the necessary internal secretion for masculine development. Lydston acquired testicles from an accident victim and fifty-four hours later performed the implant. More than likely, the testicles were implanted in the lower abdomen because of the infantile scrotum. During the recovery period, the patient gained weight and, astonishingly, after eight weeks began to have what Lydston described as "frequent and violent erections." Even more incredible was the announcement some weeks later that the man married and was reported to have "sustained the marital relation satisfactory to both parties." Lydston does not document whether the man began to shave, experienced a lowering of his voice, or developed pubic hair. Much about this case is highly questionable. And were the results of Lydston's other cases exaggerated? A number of the cases he reported were on the edge of believability. In his enthusiasm to promote gland surgery, he stretched reality. Perhaps Lydston was seeking "the minds that must be struck hard," to quote Claude Bernard.

Late in his career, Lydston overstated his role in gland surgery. In 1922, he reported he was the first to "successfully transplant a testicle from one human to another."[39] Thus, he ignored the transplant performed by Hammond and Sutton in 1912, and the report of a testicle transplant by fellow Chicagoan Victor Lespinasse in 1913. Perhaps professional jealousy played a role in Lydston's overlooking Lespinasse's report. Lydston also claimed to be the first to have experimented with gland emulsions, overlooking the original report by Brown-Séquard. Lydston also maintained that cases of "imperfect sex development" were potentially curable by sex gland implantation.[40] It's not clear what Lydston meant by this statement, but it covers such a wide variety of situations that, before modern genetics and endocrine studies which today can provide accurate diagnoses, Lydston's claim is pure speculation.

Lydston retired in 1920, and he and his wife moved to California, the state of his boyhood home. In 1923, Lydston contracted pneumonia and died on March 14. His death notice in the *Journal of the American Medical Association* described him as a "man of aggressive personality and a writer of ability."[41] The reference to "writer" was based on Lydston's having published several novels. Another source characterized him as a "good after dinner talker, a forceful lecturer, and an admirable and rapid operator."[42] Some of Lydston's personality was reflected in a letter written earlier in his life to his grandson. He wrote: "To sum up, I can do no better than to say with some wise if inelegant philosophy … live so that you can fearlessly look any man in the eye and tell him to go to hell."[43] This might have been Lydston's response to any man who rose to challenge his results.

Lydston's reports on testicle implantation inspired a plastic surgeon in New York, Dr. H. Lyons Hunt, to enter the field. Dr. Hunt wrote, "Lydston was the first to perform gland transplantation on human beings."[44] This statement was obviously not true. Also, a close reading of Lydston's reports would have led Hunt to use Lydston's word "implantation," instead of transplantation. Hunt maintained the medical profession acknowledged Lydston's experience "only when newspapers of the world began to give sensational reports, and they were joined in the more or less witty jokes about the matter." Hunt must have assumed the medical profession did not read the *Journal of the American Medical Association* nor the *New York Medical Journal*, the journals in which Lydston published most of his works.

In 1922, Hunt published two cases of men into whom he transplanted a testicle.[45] The first was a sixty-five-year-old man who became impotent following a "sudden mental shock." Hunt didn't define the shock. The man partially recovered sexual function, with the aid of "strychnine and glandular extract," only to suffer a second shock and a return of impotence. Hunt made no mention of any psychiatric evaluation. He evaluated the man and determined he could rejuvenate him with a testicle implant. Hunt proceeded with a testicle implant, using a ram's testicle obtained from the Armour Meat Company. The gland was implanted in the "lower abdominal wall."[46] Nine days later, the patient began to experience morning erections, but by the twentieth day after surgery, the implanted testicle was observed to be sloughing out, eventually leaving only a shell of the gland. Eventually, healing was complete, and surprisingly, the man began to enjoy a "normal sex life." However, about a year later, the patient requested a reduction in the fee for surgery, claiming "he felt that his entire improvement or at least a greater part of it was psychological."[47] Hunt didn't comment whether he did or didn't reduce his fee, nor did he comment on the placebo effect related by the patient.

The next case was that of a sixty-five-year-old retired sailor who had noted a gradual onset of "debility" and impotence. Based on what Hunt believed to have been a successful outcome of his previous case, Hunt chose to implant a ram's testicle in the sailor. Hunt never specified how the testicle was sterilized. Postoperatively, the sailor developed a fever and swollen abdomen. As in the previous patient, sloughing of the implant occurred and lasted for about three weeks. Finally, after healing was complete, the sailor slowly regained his strength and was able to discard his cane. He also began to have morning erections. Hunt's appraisal of this case was that the general condition and "cerebration" of the sailor was so improved that "only a biased mentality could think of denying the benefits of the testicular gland." He made no reference to the stormy postoperative course suffered by both men.

Hunt updated his transplant experience in 1923, claiming to have performed eighty-four procedures.[48] He cited the use of ovaries and testicles in his gland practice, and claimed only eight failures. Some of these cases were quite remarkable. One was that of a thirty-nine-year-old woman who had suffered such severe menstrual cramps that, on various occasions, she required chloroform, ether, or morphine for pain relief. Hunt didn't explain if these agents were used monthly or only when the pain was particularly severe. In an effort to relieve the painful symptoms, Hunt was asked to evaluate the patient for a possible ovarian transplant, which he agreed to perform. The operation was apparently a success, because several months later, the lady wrote to Hunt that the transplant "appears more in the light of a miracle to one who suffered the pains of child birth each month for twenty-five years."[49] Hunt did not specify if the menstrual pains began after a painful childbirth or if the woman only imagined what labor pains were like.

In the treatment of impotence, Hunt claimed a 90 percent success rate.[50] He cited the case of a clergyman who responded favorably to a testicle implant. Presumably, Hunt was still a customer of the Armour company. In this case, the healing was complete in two weeks. The clergyman later wrote to Hunt: "Passion [was] asserting itself," and, in summary, "my vitality, nerve force, and mental action are wonderfully increased, and I feel that many years have been returned to me." This appraisal of the transplant ranks among the best yet, a complete rejuvenation.

But as time passed, Hunt became aware of the skepticism directed at those doctors who transplanted testicles. He wrote: "Gland transplantation has been ridiculed, held up to censure. It has been made the food for salacious jokes, of caustic facetiousness and of ludicrous contempt."[51] But this criticism didn't cause any introspection, and Hunt continued on his gland-transplanting quest. By 1925, Hunt claimed to have performed over three hundred transplants. However, at this point, he conceded his results were not always successful for the condition for which the transplant was performed. To him, success could mean improvement in one or more categories: overall health, mentality, vision and hearing, muscle strength, peripheral nerve function, and sexual function. The main reason for the transplant was not always included in his appraisal of success.

Hunt could be quite persistent in treating impotence, if at first the transplant was unsuccessful. When evaluating his failures, he came up with the bizarre idea of giving a "prostate extract" to augment the effect of the transplanted testicle.[52] He convinced the Eli Lilly Company to prepare such an extract. To illustrate the use of this extract, Hunt described a fifty-seven-year-old man, who became impotent after prostate surgery. Hunt had previously performed four testicle transplants in this patient, which were unsuccessful. Rams were the donors in two, bulls in the other two. Hunt did claim that the patients experienced renewed vigor and mental activity after these procedures. Finally, Hunt performed a fifth transplant, along with an injection of the prostate extract, and achieved success. This success led Hunt to claim with his added prostate injection, "There was not one case that did not show a return of sexual function."[53] Hunt certainly had credulous patients.

Hunt took pride in his clientele. These included a Harvard graduate, a surgeon in New York City, a faculty member at a New York medical school, a medical editor, two other doctors, and two wives of physicians. Obviously, education was no deterrent to those seeking rejuvenation by Dr. Hunt.

There doesn't seem to be any writings to indicate Lydston recognized Hunt's flattery that he, Lydston, was the first to perform testicle transplant surgery.[54] Lydston died the year Hunt published the article with this claim, so it is unlikely Lydston was aware of it. Had Lydston lived a few more years, he would very likely have found Hunt's results as astounding as his own.

Lydston's self-experimentation and self-surgery are in the same category as a number of reported self-experiments.[55] But they didn't make the "top ten," most likely because there was no scientific breakthrough or any benefit from placing a testicle in himself. Some self-experiments, such as the first attempt at cardiac catheterization, led the way to techniques used today in the diagnoses and treatment of a variety of cardiac diseases. In 1929, a young German intern, Werner Forssman, performed the insertion of a thin tubing (ureteral catheter) into a vein in his arm and passed it to the level of his heart. An X-ray taken at the time confirmed that the tip of the tube was in his heart.[56] Many years later, in 1956, Forssman shared the Nobel Prize in Medicine, along with André Cournand and Dickinson W. Richards, for the development of cardiac catheterization. Alas, Lydston's experiment never gained Nobel status.

As far as self-surgery goes, it's hard to top the operations performed by Dr. Even O'Neil Kane on himself. Dr. Kane performed an appendectomy on himself under local anesthesia in 1921.[57] He had performed nearly four thousand appendectomies in his career and felt quite qualified to do the procedure. Several associates were present in the operating room in the event there was a problem. His recovery was speedy. This was two years after he had amputated one of his fingers because of an infection. Then, in 1932, he performed an inguinal hernia repair on himself, again under local anesthesia.[58] Healing was uneventful. Both these operations were carried out in the semi-sitting position with the aid of a nurse and mirror. He was seventy years old when this last operation was performed. Thirty-six hours later he was up and assisting a colleague in surgery. Unfortunately, he died from pneumonia a year later.[59] No doubt there have been other self-surgeries performed over the years that weren't reported in the newspapers. But these procedures may not have carried the risk of bowel damage or blood vessel perforation, as did the procedures performed by Dr. Kane. Dr. Kane gave no particular reason for doing the surgery on himself other than he thought he was a competent surgeon, and he wanted to demonstrate this operation could be done under local anesthesia.

Lydston would have admired him.

4

Dr. Leo Leonidas Stanley
West Coast Offense

"In the last two years, the reading public has become pretty well accustomed to the almost continuous hysterical manifestations of concern for its glandular welfare.... The world is certainly in a turbulent state concerning the matter of rejuvenation...."
—Van Buren Thorne, 1922

Dr. Leo Stanley stood beneath the gallows at San Quentin Prison awaiting the arrival of the prisoner to be executed. He watched as the convicted murderer was led to the gallows, painted a robin's-egg blue, and up the thirteen steps, one step for each jury member and one for the judge.[1] The executioner placed a black hood over the prisoner's head and a noose around his neck, with the knot directed over the shoulder rather than the back of the head so as to bring about a more effective fatal dislocation of the cervical spine. The rope used for the noose had been attached to a two-hundred-pound weight for several weeks to reduce elasticity, thus preventing the body from bouncing up and down when the trap door opened, sending the convict on a fatal descent. Even with these measures to ensure a rapid death, the cessation of breathing and heartbeat could take several agonizing minutes. Following the absence of vital signs, as determined by Dr. Stanley, the body was taken to a laboratory where an autopsy was performed. This was standard practice at San Quentin following an execution unless a family member claimed the body and did not want it disturbed in any way.

Dr. Stanley did not savor his role in pronouncing a prisoner dead when he took the position as a physician at San Quentin in 1913. He had reservations about capital punishment, even when the most vicious criminals were faced with execution.[2] But he found that in death the murderer could be of some use to society. The autopsy provided anatomical specimens for use in medical research. For example, Dr. Herbert Evans, at the University of California, received testicles which he studied in an effort to define sperm production.[3] Dr. Walter Alvarez, also at the University of California, received samples of stomach and bowel for study of the motility of these structures. In one of Dr. Alvarez's reports in the *American Journal of Physiology*, he credited Dr. Stanley with providing the specimens used in his research.[4] Dr. Alvarez moved on to a distinguished career at the Mayo Clinic, and became a well-known medical journalist. Dr. Howard Naffzinger, also at the University of California, received various organs from the autopsies at San Quentin, which were important in his research.[5] He later became chairman of the department of surgery. Thus, the bodies of those executed at San Quentin played a valuable role in the development of medical science in the Bay Area.

Dr. Stanley and his wife arrived at San Quentin in 1913. The path there was not without difficulties. During his undergraduate time at Stanford University, his father, a physician in the small community of San Miguel, California, died, leaving Leo short of the funds provided by his father to continue his education. As a result, he took a job as a peanut vendor on the Southern Pacific Railroad to earn enough money to complete his undergraduate education.[6] He hoped to follow in his father's footsteps as a doctor. After returning to Stanford, he applied to and was accepted at Cooper Medical School, which later became Stanford University Medical School. To earn his tuition as a medical student, he waited on tables in the dining room and worked part time in the physiology laboratory. Shortly before graduation, he married a young lady who was a secretary in the physiology department. Upon graduation, Dr. Stanley began an internship at Lane Hospital in San Francisco. There he encountered a variety of diseases and witnessed death from many causes.

Dr. Stanley had anticipated practicing medicine in a small town, similar to the one in which he was raised. However, near the end of his internship, he became aware of the opportunity to serve as a physician at San Quentin Prison, in nearby San Rafael. The seventy-five-dollar monthly wage, plus housing, seemed like a good opportunity to earn money in a challenging setting before setting up a practice sometime in the future.[7] Dr. Stanley applied for and was accepted for the position at San Quentin, only to discover his wife had tuberculosis, a disease that would eventually claim her life. The couple decided to stay at San Quentin, believing the fresh air from nearby San Francisco Bay would hasten her recovery.

Early in his career, Dr. Stanley became aware of the first reports of testicle transplantation, and in particular, the articles by Dr. Frank Lydston.[8] After reading Lydston's indications and technique for the implants, Stanley concluded that certain prisoners, especially those about to go on parole, might benefit from the procedure. He believed that to improve the prisoners' mentation and physical strength, and in some cases restore their sexual function, were worthwhile goals. In other words, the prisoner would be rejuvenated, a concept endorsed by the warden, John E. Boyle, a reform-minded ex-newspaperman. Stanley believed the testicle graft would "turn out a man from prison in better shape than when they came in."[9]

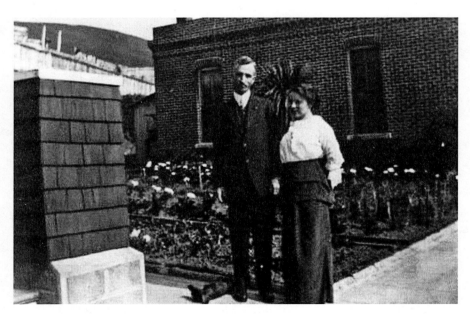

Dr. and Mrs. Stanley outside their quarters at San Quentin. At the time, Mrs. Stanley had already contracted tuberculosis and would die from the disease a decade later. (Photograph courtesy of Anne T. Kent California Reading Room, Marin County Free Library, San Rafael, California.)

4. *Dr. Leo Leonidas Stanley*

In August 1918, a twenty-seven-year-old "negro" was to be executed. Stanley believed that a prisoner, James Thompson, age twenty-five, would benefit from the testicle transplant, using the glands from the recently executed convict. Thompson had been kicked in the scrotum when he was twenty, leaving him with testicles the size of "olive pits." Thompson was described by Stanley and the prison staff as suffering from "mental and physical languor," presumably the result from the injury to his testicles.[10]

Following the execution, the testicles were removed during the autopsy and implanted in Thompson's scrotum. Three months later, Thompson was described as "considerably improved physically, mentally, and sexually." He claimed frequent erections, which he had not experienced since the injury five years earlier. In June 1919, Mr. Thompson, while on parole, was sent to a sawmill, where his work was described as "very satisfactory." In April 1920, Thompson was examined by Dr. Stanley, who described the implanted testicles as "cherry pits."[11] But the beneficial effects remained, despite the shrinkage of the glands. Thompson claimed he felt "quite energetic" and the sexual function remained during this period. Very likely the act of getting out of prison on parole played a large part in the prisoner's improvement.

Dr. Stanley's first case of testicle transplantation was included in a 1918 publication by Dr. Lydston, which included eight new cases of Lydston's. Stanley had corresponded with Lydston about his surgical technique and Lydston was flattered that Stanley had used his method. Lydston wrote: "The ... case is especially gratifying to me because the operation was performed by another surgeon."[12]

There were three or four executions at San Quentin every year in that era and Stanley used the testicles from the executed criminals in his next cases.[13] The second case was a fifty-year-old man who had suffered from inflammation of the testicles (mumps orchitis) years before, resulting in impaired sexual function. This condition was thought to have contributed to the prisoner's divorce prior to incarceration. Stanley reasoned that a new testicle would restore normal sexual function and increase the chances of the prisoner's remarrying after he had served his imprisonment. Consequently, this convict was the recipient of a testicle from an executed prisoner. Stanley usually mentioned the race or nationality of the executed donor. Five days after the surgery, the recipient experienced an erection and claimed to be having them nightly, which he had not experienced prior to the transplant. However, about six months later, he reported decreased sexual desire and frequency of erections. Dr. Stanley examined the man and found the transplanted gland had decreased to the size of a cherry. Two months later, the prisoner was induced to having the testicle removed and examined by a pathologist. The pathologist reported, "The testicle is entirely necrotic, the necrosis involving all epithelium and connective tissue. Some cellular presence was noted in the necrotic capsule."[14] Obviously, there could not have been any hormone secreted by what remained from the testicle. But Stanley was not discouraged by this finding and continued in his attempt to rejuvenate the convicts at San Quentin.

Stanley's third case was a fifty-four-year-old man who had noted declining libido and mental languor following "traumatic orchitis," four years prior to incarceration.[15] This prisoner underwent a double transplant from a "white man." Four days later the inmate experienced an erection and ejaculation. Stanley provided no further follow-up.

Case four was a seventy-two-year-old man convicted for "lascivious behavior with a minor."[16] The sex of the minor and nature of the "lascivious behavior" were not provided. Why a testicle transplant would be performed on such an individual is an obvious question. Stanley may have decided that the new gland would reorient the convict's sexual behavior. Also, the convict had been in and out of the prison infirmary on numerous occasions and Stanley thought a new gland would improve the convict's health. Subsequently, a testicle transplant was performed, using testicles from an executed Native American. On the third day after surgery, the inmate experienced an erection and was reported as having them over a ten-month period. During the immediate postoperative period, some sloughing occurred from the incision, but the incision eventually healed. Stanley made no mention of any further tendency on the part of the inmate toward "lascivious behavior" while in prison, nor was there any mention of repeat visits to the infirmary.

Stanley reported a large series of testicle transplants in 1920.[17] In this series, he included the results using ram testicles. The problem of sloughing of the transplanted glands was still encountered, but Stanley did not indicate he would discontinue the use of animal glands. Because there were too few executions to satisfy the number of candidates, he continued to use ram testicles. It is not clear if Stanley was aware of the research of Alexis Carrel, who had demonstrated that there is an immunological barrier when organs are transplanted from one species to another. In this 1920 paper, Stanley conceded that the transplanted gland was eventually doomed to failure when he wrote in the "comment" section: "We do not believe that the implant lives.... Probably in the process of necrosis, certain bodies are given off into the lymphatics of the blood stream which stimulate the patient in some unknown way."[18] Thus he no longer believed the transplant gained function and continued to secrete a hormone for a number of years. He also emphasized that the procedure did not guarantee longevity, but resulted in "good health and vigor ... and pleasure in living." This might very well contribute to a longer life.

While Stanley believed all the prisoners who underwent a testicle implant demonstrated initial improvement, he noted some experienced a relatively rapid decline in the rejuvenating effect from the operation. Another problem was that of sloughing of the gland through the incision. Consequently, he began to implant part of the gland in the abdominal wall, similar to the technique Dr. Victor Lespinasse employed. The testicles Stanley used were, at times, stored at 12°C for up to eight days, and Stanley believed the results using these glands were as good as those using fresh material.[19] This fit with his concept that the testicle eventually underwent necrosis, so time wasn't critical in the survival of the gland. He didn't record if he ever submitted one of the eight-day-old testicles to a pathologist to see how viable they appeared.

Eventually, Stanley concluded that preparing an emulsion of the testicle and injecting it would be easier than transplantation. The problem of sloughing would be eliminated, and since the testicle underwent necrosis and was eventually absorbed, the emulsion would be just as effective. Rather than grind up the gland and inject a paste-like material, Stanley cut the testicle into very small strips and injected this through a large-bore needle, the force of the injection disrupting the pieces of testicle to some extent.[20] From January 1920 to February 1922, one thousand injections were made in six hundred sixty-six prisoners. Stanley expanded the animal sources of the glands by including "goats, rams, boars, and deer," and concluded there was "very little difference in their effects...."[21] He made the point that the treatment was "fully explained and the prisoner was allowed to use his own judgment as to whether he cared to submit or not."[22] And he apparently did not offer the prisoner his choice of animal donor. Stanley never mentioned that submitting to the injections might shorten their stay in prison.

Because of the ease of administering injections, Stanley expanded his indications for use of the testicular emulsion. These included general asthenia, poor appetite, lack of energy, poor sleep habits, being underweight, and feeling "all run down."[23] It is not surprising that being incarcerated would bring on some of these complaints. Stanley noted that within a week after receiving a rejuvenating injection, convicts experienced increased appetite, weight gain, and a general "buoyancy," a term Frank Lydston used to describe his response to the implantation of a testicle in himself.[24] This term may have stuck in Stanley's mind as he was evaluating the prisoners' responses.

The injections became increasingly popular among the inmates, as was described by a reporter from the *Oakland Tribune*, who visited San Quentin looking for a story: "In this cement lined cloister, from thirty to fifty men are on the waiting list [for the injections]. Increased appetite, added vigor, greater nervous energy, and a bright outlook on life resulted from the [procedure], according to the testimony from the convicts themselves."[25] Stanley couldn't have asked for a more enthusiastic endorsement.

Thirteen physicians (not convicts) submitted to the injections.[26] Details are lacking as to what were the indications. Were they curious about what the effects might be, or did they have specific complaints which they thought might be treatable? Of interest, Stanley never admitted to injecting himself with one of the above mentioned animal sources. Perhaps he simply didn't want to be a guinea pig, as was Frank Lydston.

Early in his study of the testicular injections, Stanley considered sexual stimulation might be an endpoint by which to evaluate the effectiveness of the testicular treatment.[27] Among those inmates noting a loss of libido (Stanley used the term sexual lassitude), 85 percent experienced erotic dreams and frequent erections after treatment. Among those who were impotent without loss of libido, 65 percent responded to treatment. There were three inmates who claimed impotence after the injections, but they must have had some degree of sexual dysfunction prior to the injection to qualify for the study. The prisoners' own observation was the endpoint, and the reliability of their conclusions was open to question. Stanley did note that those receiving the injections and having some benefit told others, thus expanding the number of subjects and confirming the impression of the Oakland newspaper reporter cited earlier.

Stanley continued to expand the indications for using the testicular emulsion.[28] No longer was he using it to rejuvenate inmates about to be paroled. He now treated those with asthma, acne vulgaris (noted in young offenders), senility, dementia praecox (schizophrenia), psychopathic inferiority(?), and tuberculosis. Although he initially thought tuberculosis responded to the treatment, he later abandoned this practice. He didn't mention if he ever treated his wife with any glandular injection, as her health gradually deteriorated during this time. Another impression of Stanley's gland illusion was that young men with acne benefited from the injections, but he never stopped to consider that improved hygiene and diet in prison very likely contributed to the improvement. Often the young inmates came from impoverished conditions. Then too, many of the young inmates simply outgrew the condition.

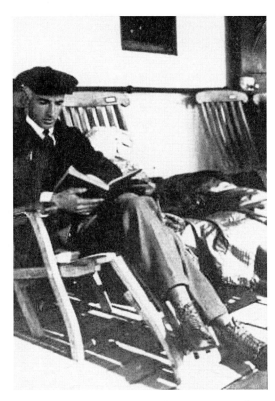

Dr. Stanley relaxing in what appears to be a deck chair, possibly on his way to San Francisco by ferryboat. (Courtesy of the Anne T. Kent California Reading Room, Marin County Free Library.)

It is unlikely that Frank Lydston's research on the use of injections from glands, organs, and other structures in the human body was of any benefit to Stanley. Lydston admitted to Stanley that his series of injections was a failure.[29] But Lydston acknowledged that

The Gland Illusion

Stanley's use of relatively fresh testicles, untreated with antiseptic and not stored for any length of time, might be effective. Stanley used testicles (obtained from a butcher) promptly, and usually made the emulsion and injections relatively soon. Apparently, Lydston was not aware that Stanley had implanted a testicle stored for eight days.

Stanley soon gained some degree of notoriety from his publications. He presented his results at a meeting of the California Medical Society in 1920. His presentation was well attended, but the following year, a representative from the Society informed Stanley that his talk had generated considerable controversy and he would not be invited to speak at the meeting next year. The representative from the Society conceded that when Dr. Stanley presented his paper, the attendance at the urology section rose from twenty-five the previous year to over a hundred. However, some members of the Society now regarded Dr. Stanley—along with Dr. John Brinkley, the Kansas "goat gland doctor" who had visited Los Angeles in 1920 and performed a number of goat testicle transplants; and Dr. Clayton Wheeler, a purveyor of goat serum made from special goats on Catalina Island—as quacks.[30] This was not the first time Stanley suspected he might be linked with quacks, and it should have prompted him to be more critical of his work. He expressed a fear of the quack label when he received an invitation from a local Kiwanis Club to give a talk on the "interstitial glands" (testicles). Stanley accepted the invitation but added, "Would you be kind enough to refrain from giving [the talk] publicity?"[31] No doubt he feared an adverse response to the announcement of his talk. Then, in 1922, Stanley published a paper in which he wrote: "In presenting this phase of the study of internal secretions, one cannot be unmindful of the publicity which has been given the interstitial gland during these past few years, and the bad impression this has made upon the medical world.... The public, however, clamored for more news about this wonderful and all-absorbing topic, with its mystery and sex-appeal. It became a very interesting subject of conversation among men and women in all walks of life."[32]

But support for Dr. Stanley came from Professor Roy Hoskins, a physiologist at Ohio State University. Hoskins wrote an editorial in the relatively new medical journal *Endocrinology* which stated: "The clinical studies, especially of Lydston and Stanley, have led to promising results.... The difficulties confronting students in this field (endocrinology) have been grossly underestimated and much paper and ink have been wasted in the promulgation of immature or even fantastic literature which the actual known facts by no means justify."[33] This statement reflected the lack of objectivity and healthy speculation that helped perpetuate the gland illusions of this era. However, it provided enough encouragement so that Stanley continued his work rejuvenating the convicts of San Quentin.

At some point in the early nineteen-twenties, Stanley was visited by Dr. Serge Voronoff from Paris, who was implanting monkey testicles in men seeking rejuvenation and increased longevity. Stanley recalled Voronoff "seemed greatly impressed" by his experience at San Quentin. Voronoff had exclaimed in his French accent, "Your operations are for zee poor man and mine are for zee rich man!"[34] It was Stanley's impression that Voronoff charged the equivalent of between five and six thousand dollars for his operation. As will be shown in a later chapter, Voronoff hardly needed the money.

Stanley's wife's health continued to deteriorate from tuberculosis until she died in 1926. He then took some time off, leaving the medical duties at San Quentin to an assistant. Upon returning to San Quentin, he began an investigation on the effect of the testicular injections on diabetes mellitus.[35] The results showed that after the injections, the sugar in the urine decreased; however, the diet and amount of exercise, two important factors in controlling diabetes, were not closely regulated. Hence, it was not proven that the injections were responsible for any improvement in the diabetic condition of the inmates in the study. The subsequent discovery of insulin discouraged any further experiments in treating diabetes using a testicular product.

When there was an execution, the testicles obtained at autopsy continued to be used for transplantation. In 1928, a death sentence was carried out on a murderer, Charles L. "Buck" Kelly. Kelly and an accomplice had gone on a robbing and killing spree. The pair were quickly apprehended, tried and sentenced to death by hanging.[36] Prior to the execution, Kelly had inquired whether an autopsy would be performed. Stanley informed him that autopsies were routinely done to collect information of value for medical science. On hearing this, Kelly gave a "contemptuous laugh" and told Stanley they could have his brain and "cremate the rest of me…. I am a con and my old man is a con."[37] Kelly's father was also a prisoner at San Quentin, having been convicted for

robbery, and was confined to the mental ward known as "crazy alley."
Many autopsies had been done at San Quentin over the years, and Dr.
Stanley assumed this was standard practice. But he subsequently discovered that after death, the body belongs to the next of kin, and a
prisoner cannot will his body for science without the family's permission.

On the day of the execution, Stanley noted a certain swagger to
Buck as he approached the gallows. Buck seemed "flattered" by the
crowd gathered to witness the execution.[38] The crime had been one of
the more sensational in recent history in the Bay Area. Kelly was led
up the scaffold, and as the executioner applied the noose and placed a
black hood over his head, Stanley heard him call out like a frightened
child, "Good-by mother."[39] Kelly's poor mother was waiting on the other
side of the bay for the fatal hour, after which she would set out for the
mortuary to claim the body.

Following the execution, an autopsy was performed by Dr. W.T.
Cummings.[40] From the autopsy, one testicle was sent to Dr. Hans Liss-
ner at the University of California for study, and the other was sent to
the University of California Hospital for implantation in an older
patient considered a candidate for rejuvenation.[41] A newspaper reporter,
I.P. McDowell, had followed Kelly's body to the mortuary and was
allowed to view it. He noted an autopsy had been performed and the
scrotum appeared empty. The reporter did not divulge whether he
knew or suspected that the testicles would be removed, but the next
day, the reporter filed a story containing the inflammatory headline:
"Kelly Mutilated."[42] The story revealed that a testicle transplant was
performed in a San Francisco hospital, the name and location not given.
In an effort to quiet the uproar the story created, the *San Francisco
Examiner* published an editorial trying to put the event in perspective:
"The valuable and progressive work done for medical science under
the auspices of Dr. L.L. Stanley, the San Quentin physician, ought not
to be interrupted because of the Buck Kelly autopsy.... Failure to obtain
a family consent was, of course, an irregularity and such irregularities
should not occur. But in the other column must be recorded the many
years of remarkable work done at San Quentin for the benefit of human
suffering."[43]

While this editorial quieted public concerns, Buck's mother sued
the prison medical staff, and eventually a "nuisance award" was paid.

4. Dr. Leo Leonidas Stanley

Months later, Dr. Stanley reflected on the Buck Kelly event and sympathized with Mrs. Kelly. He had witnessed her in her worn, shabby coat visiting San Quentin, sometimes bringing a small gift for Buck or her husband. To Stanley, she represented "all the stricken mothers of men who have been hanged.... He was still the core of his mother's heart and she could still find pride in him."[44] Finally, Dr. Stanley was made aware of the fact that a person who is executed "cannot will his remains to a person or organization. Only the next of kin has the right to make such a disposal."[45] Many times, there were no relatives available or willing to claim the body, but in Buck's case, his mother would have been the one to give permission. The testicle from Buck Kelly sent to the University of California Hospital was implanted into an elderly man who felt so "invigorated" that he sexually attacked a nurse. The patient was brought to trial and convicted of rape.[46] His fate was that he was sent to San Quentin. Thus the testicle from Buck Kelly made a round trip from San Quentin to the patient in the hospital and back to San Quentin.

In this era, there was an attempt to link criminality with "abnormal glands."[47] Dr. Stanley and Dr. Arthur Reynolds, a San Francisco physician, concluded that "murderers in San Quentin have abnormal glands (referring to all glands) ... that every social misfit displayed malsecretion of some gland." Dr. Reynolds went on to say, "One youthful convicted slayer ... attacked other prisoners and has an abnormal thyroid gland upon which we operated and reduced to what we thought [was normal] and today the prisoner is entirely tractable. Sixty other inmates were treated in this manner." No mention was made about how permission was obtained, either from the warden or the inmate. This news was picked up by *Time* magazine, which published an article titled "Criminal Glands."[48] The conclusion of the article was that surgery, or treatment with "glandular extracts" suggested a way of "reforming criminals." There was no follow-up on this series of glandular interventions. It is possible that an inmate who was hyperthyroid would benefit from a reduction in the size of the thyroid. And there may have been convicts in whom reducing the size of the thyroid made them more docile (hypothyroid) and easier to control. But Stanley doesn't provide any long-term results and the interest in "criminal glands" gradually disappeared.

Another project initiated by Dr. Stanley was voluntary sterilization.

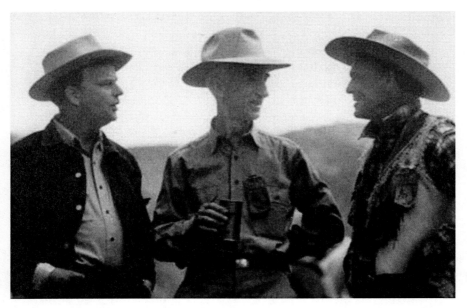

Dr. Stanley is in the center of this photograph, flanked on the left by the famous ventriloquist Edgar Bergen, and on his right by Dick Dixon. The photograph was taken in 1947. (Courtesy of the Anne T. Kent California Reading Room, Marin County Free Library.)

In 1935 he posted a notice in the prison yard informing the inmates about vasectomy.[49] In addition to sterilization, Stanley advanced the concept that occluding the vas deferens might improve one's health. This idea was promoted by Professor Eugen Steinach in Vienna, and Dr. Harry Benjamin in New York. Steinach's research will be discussed in a later chapter. Stanley was careful to clear this project with the attorney general of California. Among the reasons why an inmate might want to have a vasectomy were these: don't want children or don't want more children added to their family after discharge from prison; don't want children to carry the stigma of having a convict or ex-convict as a father; and to improve their health. One hundred twenty-six prisoners subsequently signed up for the procedure.[50] This was during the depression, and the cost of raising a child undoubtedly influenced some convicts to want to avoid fathering a child. How long this project lasted was not revealed in Stanley's memoir.

After Stanley's wife died, he began to take more time off from his prison duties. During these breaks, he served as a physician on passenger ships of the Matson line.[51] He remarried in 1938, and the couple settled first in San Rafael, then in nearby Fairfax. After the Pearl Harbor attack and the United States' entry into World War II, Dr. Stanley enlisted in the Navy and served on several hospital ships until the end of hostilities. He then resumed his duties at San Quentin until he retired in 1951.[52] The gland rejuvenation project had faded away long before his retirement. Stanley never pinpointed when he no longer felt the need to rejuvenate some of the inmates at San Quentin.

Dr. Stanley served as physician at San Quentin for thirty-seven years and earned the title of "Chief Croaker," among the inmates.[53] Upon retiring, he practiced medicine in San Rafael for several years, then became involved in the activities of the San Rafael water district. He wrote several histories of the San Rafael area, and of San Miguel, where his family had lived when he was a boy.

Dr. Stanley became an avid horseman, and he and his wife belonged to several riding clubs in the San Rafael area. In addition to these activities, the couple maintained a sizable garden in their ten-acre estate in Fairfax.[54]

During Dr. Stanley's travels, he occasionally encountered former inmates. Once, while in Mexico, he was hailed by a man who had been treated by Stanley for some condition, at San Quentin. This former inmate, plus others living in the area who had been former inmates at San Quentin, showed the "greatest cordiality" toward Stanley.[55] In Sydney, Australia, Stanley met "two of our boys [who] offered to show me the sights of the city."[56] At Lake Tahoe, he was hailed by a former prisoner who was accompanied by "three or four ladies." The man exclaimed, "Look, here is Dr. Stanley, the man who rejuvenated me." Stanley suspected this former prisoner had undergone a testicle implant or injection of the testicular emulsion and he was a bit unnerved by this enthusiastic greeting.[57]

Dr. Leo Stanley died on November 13, 1976.[58] He was remembered not just for the gland experiments but for establishing a tuberculosis ward, which decreased the incidence of this disease at San Quentin. He was also recognized for his expertise in spinal anesthesia. When he arrived at San Quentin, he found the individual providing general anesthesia had a weakness for laboratory alcohol and was unreliable, even dangerous.[59] Since the majority of surgical procedures performed at

San Quentin only required anesthesia below the waist, spinal anesthesia was effective and could be administered by Dr. Stanley himself.

Stanley was also recognized for his work in plastic surgery. Many of the convicts bore facial scars from previous altercations and wished to have them corrected while in prison. One such example was a prisoner nicknamed "Wolf," because of his lupine facial features. The prisoner feared his appearance would frighten people when he was paroled. Stanley corrected his features such that, as a reporter for the *San Francisco Examiner* described the result of the surgery, the "face would have passed Little Red Riding Hood's closest scrutiny."[60] Another of Stanley's contributions to plastic surgery was a technique for correcting a deformed broken nose by refracturing it and realigning the cartilage and nasal bones. This technique was published in *Surgery Gynecology & Obstetrics* (now the *Journal of the American College of Surgeons).*[61] All in all, Dr. Stanley did turn out many men better than when they entered prison.

Today, the prison population across the United States is considerably different from that in Dr. Stanley's era. No longer is tuberculosis a major health problem as it was in the past, but instead hypertension, diabetes, hepatitis, HIV infection and mental health problems, including drug addiction, are major challenges for those caring for convicts.[62] No amount of gland therapy would help these medical conditions.

5

Dr. Serge Voronoff and Monkey Glands

"There is every reason that the existing folly will follow in the footsteps of the past ... and will drop from public view like a fruit which has ripened into spontaneous rottenness...."
—Dr. Oliver Wendell Holmes

The chimpanzee was netted in its cage and transferred to a small wooden box just large enough to hold the animal. The sides of the box were closed except for a small opening in the top to observe the chimp, and another small opening through which ethyl chloride was dripped into the box. When the chimp appeared drowsy enough to handle safely, the box was opened quickly and the animal placed on an operating table and the limbs secured. Chloroform was then administered to provide complete anesthesia.[1]

On another operating table in the same surgical suite, Dr. Serge Voronoff placed a fifty-five-year-old man in position for surgery on his scrotum. Both the patient and the chimp underwent shaving of the lower abdomen and genitalia, followed by a thorough washing of the shaved area and the application of iodine and alcohol. Following this skin preparation, Dr. George Voronoff, Serge's brother, incised the scrotum of the chimp and removed the testicles. Simultaneously, Dr. Serge Voronoff injected local anesthesia into the patient's scrotal skin. After several minutes, an incision was made in the patient's scrotum and the testicles exposed. With great care, the thin membrane (tunica vaginalis) surrounding the testicle was exposed. Dr. Serge Voronoff then divided the testicles from the chimp into several longitudinal segments, the size that would fit within the opened tunica vaginalis. Voronoff's concept behind this operation was that the secretion from the testicular

61

segments would be absorbed through the thin tunica and into the patient's circulation. The tunica was then closed over these segments, followed by closure of the skin incision. A sterile dressing was applied. Usually, the patient remained in the clinic for a few days before traveling to his home.[2]

The fifty-nine-year-old man into whom Dr. Voronoff had just implanted pieces of chimpanzee testicle had sought Voronoff's expertise because of memory loss, depression, and loss of libido.[3] He had heard of Voronoff's treatment of these symptoms in older men, supposedly making them years younger. Several months later, the patient reported that his memory had improved and he had regained "intellectual activity." However, the libido was slow to return. Voronoff usually advised waiting several months for a return

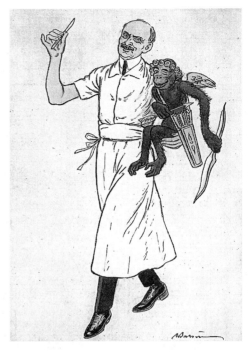

"A New Gift from Cupid." This cartoon from an Italian magazine shows Dr. Serge Voronoff, scalpel in hand, holding a monkey representing Cupid, ready to launch an arrow of love. The recipient of the arrow will probably need Dr. Voronoff's services. (From *Scena Illustrata*, April 1–15, 1927.)

of sexual function, although he had noted sexual excitement could occur relatively soon after surgery, only to dissipate for a period of time. Voronoff's observation that sexual activity could occur soon after the transplant was not too different from that of Lespinasse and Lydston.

How Serge Voronoff came to the practice of transplantating primate testicles in men is a unique story. Voronoff was born in Russia in 1866.[4] After he and his brothers emigrated from Russia to France, Serge attended medical school in Paris, graduating in 1885. Subsequently, he became a French citizen to facilitate obtaining a position in which to practice medicine. To achieve clinical experience, he accepted a position in the Royal Court of Egypt, a position that had been recommended by his instructors in medical school. While in Egypt, he observed eunuchs in the royal court. He appraised them as being intellectually slow and lacking courage and enterprise. They "grew old before their time."[5] In Voronoff's mind, the eunuchs resembled old men. Hence, it was not unreasonable for him to conclude that a product from the testicle would rejuvenate older men suffering from the effects of aging.

Voronoff returned to France in 1912, where he turned his attention to female infertility. Voronoff and his wife had no children and this may have stimulated his interest in infertility. He was also intrigued by the pioneering research of Dr. Alexis Carrel in organ transplantation.[6] He initiated correspondence with Carrel, hoping to gain insight into Carrel's experience, with the goal of transplanting ovaries to correct infertility. Voronoff's letters indicated he had acquired a position in a research facility and had already achieved some success in transplanting ovaries into sheep.[7] Voronoff did mention that, in his brief experience, the sheep into which the ovaries were transplanted should be from the same blood line—"similar blood was needed." Thus Voronoff recognized there was an immunological barrier when transplanting ovaries from unrelated animals, a conclusion Carrel had already reached in his research in kidney transplantation. Carrel offered little encouragement for Voronoff's research.[8]

In 1914 the First World War began, and Voronoff transferred his efforts to caring for wounded soldiers. He served in a French military hospital and specialized in wound treatment. He focused on the relatively new technique of bone grafting, until his military service was terminated when he developed an infection in his arm.[9] Later that year, 1917, he and his wife divorced. Perhaps Voronoff's interest in infertility was prompted by the failure of the couple to have children. After the war, Voronoff gave up on his attempts at ovarian grafting. He wrote, "In the case of females, I have not observed any marked influence [success] from grafting."[10]

With no established medical practice, Voronoff, at the recommendation of an old teacher, obtained a position at the College de France. He would later become director of the Physiological Station at the college.[11] Thus Voronoff would follow in the path of distinguished scientists at the college, including Claude Bernard and Brown-Séquard. Voronoff must have demonstrated enough scientific promise, based on his wartime experience, to warrant this appointment.

It was Brown-Séquard who had stimulated interest in the secretion from the testicle as a source of rejuvenation. Voronoff followed this concept with the idea of transplanting a testicle from a relatively young animal into an aging animal such as a ram or goat in order to rejuvenate it.[12] He recalled his experience in Egypt, observing men in whom the reproductive glands had been removed and how they seemed to have aged prematurely. Voronoff began his experiment using rams and goats because they were of the size that allowed relatively easy observation of the transplant site and the overall appearance of the animal.[13] At first he transplanted the whole testicle, but regarded the results as unsatisfactory. Then he began to transplant segments onto the recipient's testicle, beneath the tunica vaginalis. Using this technique, he grafted segments from the testicles of young healthy rams onto the testicles of aging rams and noted that the older rams appeared healthier and more vigorous. This was a highly subjective appraisal by Voronoff, who had no formal training in veterinary medicine. And there were no control animals in whom a sham operation had been performed for comparison. What Voronoff interpreted as an improved appearance may have been due to better care after the surgery.

Voronoff then shifted his attention to goats. His surgical procedure consisted of placing segments of the donor testicle on the surface of the recipient and then closing the lining over the testicle to allow absorption of the testicular secretion to pass through the lining. To prove to himself that the transplanted testicular segments were functioning, Voronoff removed a transplanted gland after a year and had it examined by a pathologist, Édouard Retterer. The pathologist interpreted the specimen as showing the presence of live testicular cells. However, it is likely what Retterer observed was an accumulation of inflammatory cells, thus contributing to Voronoff's mistaken belief that the transplanted segments of testicle were functioning.[14]

By 1919, Voronoff had acquired enough animal data to present his results to the French Surgical Congress. The press became aware of this report about restoring youthful vigor to aging rams and goats. Voronoff was also quoted as implying "there was no reason not to do so in man."[15] Already the era of testicle transplants/implants had been initiated in the United States by Victor Lespinasse and Frank Lydston, and soon Voronoff would embark on a course of transplanting monkey testicles into humans.

Voronoff remarried in 1920. His new wife, Frances Evelyn Bostwick, had been a laboratory assistant at the college and had assisted

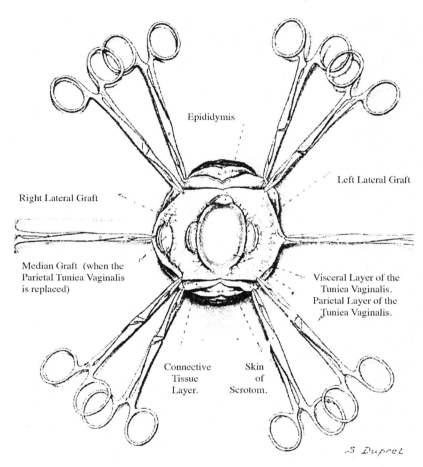

The drawing shows the location of fragments of the chimpanzee's testicle that were placed on the recipient's testicle. The thin tunica vaginalis was then closed over the gland. The thin tunica was supposed to allow the passage of the male hormone into the recipient's circulation. But the implanted segments of testicle had no blood supply, and no doubt degenerated into scar tissue. (From Serge Voronoff, *Rejuvenation by Grafting*, 1925.)

Voronoff in his early experiments.[16] She was the daughter of one of the founders of Standard Oil, and on the death of her father, she became immensely wealthy. That summer Voronoff and his new wife sailed for New York for the purpose of settling the Bostwick family estate. Voronoff's arrival in New York aroused interest in the press, who had been following the reports of Voronoff's gland transplantation. There was great speculation that Voronoff had transplanted a monkey testicle into a human. Madam Voronoff, acting as translator, denied any such procedure had been performed, but it had.[17] Later it was revealed that before departing on their trip, Voronoff had performed two transplants using chimpanzee testicles and both cases failed. The two patients suffered from tuberculosis, which had destroyed their testicles. The disease had also affected their lungs and urinary tract. If knowledge of these failures had emerged at that time, Voronoff would have faced embarrassing questions about the transplant results. In retrospect, these two patients were hardly good risks because the disease had destroyed the site into which the transplanted glands were placed.

While in New York, Voronoff performed a testicle transplant in a dog for the faculty at Columbia University College of Physicians and Surgeons.[18] Although the demonstration was carried somewhat in secret, one outsider did know about the event. This person was Dr. Max Thorek, a surgeon from Chicago, who had become interested in testicle transplantation through the influence of Dr. Frank Lydston. Thorek had wired Voronoff, requesting literature on the subject. Voronoff responded that he would be in New York and was willing to meet with Dr. Thorek to discuss the subject. Thorek and his wife did meet Voronoff and his wife for dinner at the Bostwick home in New York City. During dinner, Thorek invited Voronoff to visit Chicago and give a demonstration similar to the one at Columbia. Voronoff initially declined, but then relented and made the trip to Chicago. Thorek had hoped Voronoff would meet Lydston, who had been transplanting testicles since 1914.

Thorek returned to Chicago and arranged for a live demonstration to be held at the American Hospital.[19] Voronoff came to Chicago, and with his wife as assistant, he performed the testicle transplant in a dog, before a packed audience. Conspicuous by his absence was Frank Lydston, who purposefully avoided meeting Voronoff because of a grievance against him. Lydston felt Voronoff had avoided acknowledging the role of American doctors in the development of testicle transplantation. Thorek must have been informed that Lydston would not be attending the demonstration and informed Voronoff of Lydston's boycott. As a diplomatic gesture, Voronoff sent Lydston a note requesting his presence and recognizing his experience in implanting testicles. However, Lydston would not budge in his resentment of the Frenchman, and this resentment continued throughout Lydston's career.

After Voronoff and his wife returned to Paris, he resumed his research on testicle transplantation and rejuvenation. Although he sought human donors, he found the fee for glands too high, and obtaining glands from the recently deceased too difficult. Consequently, he chose to use testicles from chimpanzees and baboons, species closely related to humans.[20] In 1920 he performed four testicle transplants at private clinics, using primate glands.

Later in 1920, Voronoff published his book, *Life*, in French; it was later translated into English by his wife.[21] His book explained the concept of replacing a worn-out gland by transplanting a young gland (testicle) into the body, thereby rejuvenating a person and reducing the effects of aging. But Voronoff recognized there were other factors influencing the lifespan in humans. He noted that the majority of the elderly were "poor people."[22] Poverty forced an individual to lead a sober life. Such individuals are content with a diet of "bread, milk, and vegetables," and avoided excess in all things. This observation is not too dissimilar from the current concept of caloric restriction and increasing vegetable consumption to promote longevity. But in his later writings, Voronoff did not focus on these preventative measures; he was far more interested in using gland transplantation as a means of restoring mind and body.

In his book, Voronoff stressed the importance of using simian glands as a source of rejuvenation.[23] He seemed unaware of the risk of transmitting simian diseases to humans by transplanting a testicle from a chimpanzee into a human. In particular, there was a risk of transmitting what is now referred to as simian (human) immunodeficiency virus (HIV-1) to humans, the cause of AIDS.[24] Because the majority of Voronoff's patients were in their fifties and sixties, the possible emergence of AIDS might have been overlooked or attributed to the aging process.

Having established his technique for grafting segments of chimpanzee testicle to the human gland, Voronoff initiated an active program for rejuvenation. He did acknowledge that only the superficial part of the graft survived, but he concluded that what he interpreted as the surviving cells adapt to their new environment and supply the needed secretion. In the appendix to his book he stated: "It is not the interstitial cells which take charge of the internal secretion."[25] Presumably, he did not see any interstitial cells and assumed other cells were the source of the secretion. At this point in time, it was generally accepted that the interstitial cell (Leydig cell) was the source of what is now termed testosterone. Thus, Voronoff was wrong in his interpretation of the function of the transplanted cells seen under the microscope.

Reviews of a subsequent book by Voronoff on the subject of testicle transplantation, *Greffes Testiculares*, evoked adverse criticism from one reviewer. The *British Medical Journal* noted there had been an objection to Voronoff's presenting a paper at the French Congress of Surgery.[26] The objection had been based partly on a technicality, but the leader of the Congress was emphatic that the paper, which summarized Voronoff's research in gland transplantation, should not be presented.[27] Consequently, Voronoff presented his paper the next day at the College of France. According to the *New York Times*, the publicity given to this presentation attracted a large crowd of those curious to hear the results of Voronoff's research.[28] However, it was noted that Parisian surgeons and physicians were conspicuous by their absence.

Another criticism leveled at Voronoff's book was that his investigations were "exceedingly suggestive and of the greatest interest [but] ... the more skeptical scientist will demand further details before he can accept all that the author claims."[29] A far more unfavorable impression of Voronoff's research appeared in the relatively new journal *Endocrinology*. The reviewer stated: "The poor impression of this book created by the wretched illustrations and worse paper is borne out by reading the text."[30] The reviewer pointed out the biopsies of the transplanted glands showed degeneration of the sperm-producing cells and the lack of mitotic figures among the interstitial cells, indicating nonviable tissue. Another point of criticism was the erroneous concept put forth by Voronoff and Retterer, a pathologist working with Voronoff, that the interstitial (hormone-producing) cells evolved from the sperm-producing cells (spermatocytes). There were other concepts in the book which were simply incorrect. The reviewer concluded that the book "should be read very critically or, better, not at all." Voronoff's ideas seemed to have triggered considerable antagonism and contempt toward him.

Voronoff's response to the adverse criticism of his work was that there were scientists who were jealous of his work. After the French Congress of Surgery refused to hear his paper, he responded by claiming, "It was an organized attempt against me actuated by jealousy. The only thing that remains for me is to publish the results of my experiments in a book...."[31] This statement suggests his work might have been rejected by more than one scientific journal.

In 1920, Frank Lydston was mentioned in the *New York Times* as being one of the originators of testicle transplanting. This was before Voronoff had begun his research in humans.[32] Lydston never forgot how Voronoff had advanced his own career, never acknowledging the earlier reports of Lespinasse and himself. Voronoff also never cited the research of those attempting to grow cells from various organs outside the human body (in vitro). In 1911, Fleisher and Loeb reported on their attempts at growing fragments of guinea pig testicles on a blood clot, the clot being regarded as the source of nutrients for cell growth.[33] They observed cells toward the periphery of the testicular fragments survived to some extent, but there was no evidence that any of the cells grew into the clot, as tissues from some other structures in the body had been observed to do. This observation suggests that pieces of transplanted testicle may not become incorporated into surrounding tissue and establish an effective blood supply so as to maintain viability. Attention to the reports of in vitro studies might have made Voronoff more cautious in interpreting his results.

Voronoff's career could be followed in the *New York Times*. This may have been related to his marriage to Evelyn Bostwick and the gossip surrounding the settlement of the Bostwick estate. After the estate was settled, Evelyn donated considerable shares of Standard Oil stock to Voronoff's laboratory. Unfortunately, Voronoff's marriage to Evelyn was short-lived; she died in 1921, leaving him the recipient of the interest on the Bostwick investments.[34]

Even the acquisition of monkeys by Voronoff became a subject of interest, feeding the public's curiosity about his rejuvenation studies. On one occasion, the *Times* reported that Voronoff had purchased two monkeys at a street fair in Rouen.[35] Then Voronoff made news when two monkeys escaped from his laboratory.[36] To solve the problem of obtaining monkeys, Voronoff established a monkey colony near Nice.[37] This colony supplied the need for primates, which he had been importing from French colonies in Africa. Voronoff maintained this colony until the beginning of World War II, when the area was seized by Italian forces, then part of the Axis.

The degree of interest in glands by the general public was further illustrated in the popular literature of the time. In Dorothy Sayers's mystery, *The Unpleasantness at the Bellona Club*, one of the characters, Mrs. Rushworth, questions Lord Peter Wimsey, a wealthy amateur detective, about young criminals. Wimsey replies: "They presented a very perplexing problem." Mrs. Rushworth responds: "How very true. So perplexing. And to think that we have been quite wrong about them all these years. Flogging and bread and water, you know, and Holy Communion, when what they really needed was a bit of rabbit gland or something to make them good as gold."[38]

Interest in glands also attracted the attention of Arthur Conan Doyle, author of the Sherlock Holmes detective mysteries. In the story "The Adventure of the Creeping Man," Holmes is enlisted to solve the bizarre behavior of a noted professor, who has been observed climbing the side of his home.[39] When the professor is bitten by his pet dog and temporarily incapacitated, Holmes seizes the opportunity to search the professor's personal items. His search turns up an empty vial and a syringe. The vial has been sent from Prague, and a letter accompanying the vial indicated it contained serum from a "black faced langur," a monkey noted for its climbing ability. Holmes deduced that the professor had been injecting himself with this serum, leading to the propensity to climb. Further detective work revealed that the professor was a widower and had recently become attracted to a comely young woman. He hoped the serum would have a rejuvenating effect on his aging body. Holmes ended the story by sending a letter to the scientist in Prague who produced the serum, threatening criminal proceedings unless production of the serum stopped immediately. He added: "The highest type of man may revert to the animal, if he leaves the road of destiny." In other words, follow the course in life that nature intended.

In 1925, Voronoff published a book, *Rejuvenation by Grafting*, which summarized the results of forty-four cases of testicle grafting.[40] Evidence of rejuvenation included improvement in several conditions associated with aging. The most frequent indication was impotence, followed by memory loss and senility. Depression was the primary indication in 20 percent. In many of these patients there was more than one diagnosis. Slightly more than half the men undergoing a testicle transplant were deemed to have recovered their potency, although some noted only slight improvement. But a sixty-seven-year-old man claimed his sexual activity returned to an "extraordinary degree."[41] Voronoff claimed this elderly gentleman appeared fifteen years younger. Improvement in overall health was noted in a variety conditions, including constipation, tremor, leg cramps, colitis, and stroke. In some cases, improvement in overall health was noted, but the impotence, the chief reason for having the transplant, remained unchanged. Improvement in depression was documented by observing that the patient appeared "more alert, displayed increased vigor, jovial eyes, and had more energy," without actually stating that the depression had resolved.

In addition to the testicle grafting in humans, Voronoff and associates continued experiments on sheep and goats.[42] His results in grafting indicated to him that the grafting resulted in increased wool production. The animals were also reported to have gained weight, indicating increased meat production. This practice would be a boon to ranchers, and to veterinarians who would perform the testicle grafting. Voronoff also experimented with grafting a testicle from a young stallion to a retired race horse.[43] The plan was to enter the rejuvenated race horse in a contest the following year, hoping the horse would make a creditable showing. However, there was no follow-up to this venture. Instead, there was another attempt at grafting a testicle into a horse, which resulted in death.[44] The event seemed to have discouraged Voronoff from further experiments on horses. Also, horse breeders questioned the paternity of the offspring from a stallion in which part of a testicle from another horse had been grafted.

In 1925, an article by an editor of a veterinary medicine journal summarized Voronoff's results in grafting testicles in rams and goats.[45] It cited two hundred operations performed for the purpose of increasing wool production and longevity in certain animals for breeding. This article also cited Voronoff's efforts, working with Italian veterinarians, in grafting a testicle from a stallion into a mule. The goal of this surgical stunt was not provided, nor was the outcome.

Some of Voronoff's experiments with cattle, sheep, and goats were performed at an experimental farm near Algiers. By 1928, there was

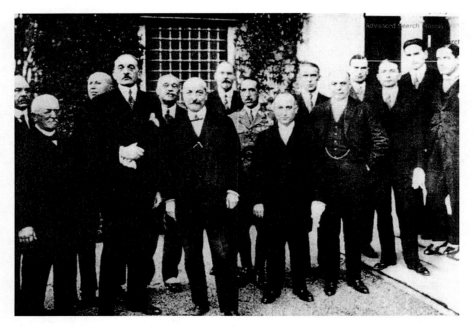

The delegation who traveled to Algeria to visit the experimental farm where Voronoff carried out his research on sheep. The delegation was not impressed with his results. Voronoff is the tall gentlemen fourth from the left. (Courtesy of the Wellcome Library, London.)

enough interest and skepticism about Voronoff's results that a delegation from the British Ministry of Agriculture, including a physiologist, geneticist, dietician, and veterinary surgeon, along with observers from other countries, visited the farm.[46] After arriving at the farm, the delegation was shown a seventeen-year-old-bull, which was reported to have been rejuvenated and subsequently sired nine calves. Ordinarily, a bull that age was past its prime as a breeding animal. When the delegation reviewed the paternity of some of the calves, there were questions about the sire. Flocks of sheep were inspected for their wool and mutton production and the pedigrees for each animal were found to be lacking. The delegation conceded that claims of rejuvenation may be valid but the evidence was not based on "critical experimentation."[47] Finally, the delegation concluded: "There is a great need for repetition of these experiments with standard material under controlled conditions of husbandry."

5. Dr. Serge Voronoff and Monkey Glands

While not condemning Voronoff's animal experiments, the British report certainly cast some doubt on the validity of his research. A far more critical and detailed study of testicle grafting in sheep emerged from a French breeding station in Morocco headed by veterinary surgeon Henri Velu.[48] Velu was aware of Voronoff's remarkable results and, with an element of suspicion, had started his own testicle-grafting project in sheep. His carefully supervised study showed no effect on wool production nor the weight of the sheep. In addition, when the implanted segments of testicle were biopsied, the results showed only scar tissue and inflammatory cells.[49] Velu presented his results at a meeting of the French Veterinary Académie in 1929, ending his talk by labeling Voronoff's claims "une grande illusion."[50] By 1931, Voronoff's Algerian sheep rejuvenation project was curtailed.

An Australian study of testicle grafting in sheep also reported negative findings.[51] The report showed no evidence of increased mutton production nor of wool production. Thus, Voronoff's grand experiment and his reputation were coming under fire.

In Germany, Dr. Hofmeister, at the University of Friburg, reported that gland transplantation was a failure.[52] Monkeys were used in his research and he found the transplanted testicles were absorbed relatively rapidly after surgery, and, although there seemed to be a temporary rejuvenation, a loss of vitality followed.

Voronoff received another setback in 1928, in addition to the negative impression of his experimental farm generated by the British report. After the death of his second wife, Evelyn Bostwick, he remarried, only to have his third wife, Louise Ignatiff, sue for divorce, claiming abandonment.[53] She complained that Voronoff spent most of his time at a miniature jungle and monkey colony near Cannes. No doubt he was working on new experiments involving glands.

A rival to Voronoff's method for rejuvenation emerged in Vienna when Dr. Karl Doppler reported on his technique for rejuvenation. It consisted of applying phenol to the artery to the testicle.[54] This was performed through an inguinal incision. The phenol was supposed to impair the sympathetic nerves overlying the artery, thus causing dilation of the artery and increasing blood flow to the testicle. In theory, the increased blood flow would result in increased output from the interstitial cells. Doppler claimed successful rejuvenation in two hundred cases. However, he told a *New York Times* reporter not to give any publicity to his work, and for that reason, he refused an invitation to lecture in America. No doubt he feared the question as to how often the phenol damaged the nerves and the underlying artery (spermatic artery) to the testicle. Controversy soon arose over the validity of Doppler's research, and he was referred to as a "bigger monkey than Voronoff."[55]

Despite mounting criticism, such was Voronoff's reputation as an expert in gland surgery that he was invited to lecture the Cambridge University Medical Society. At this meeting, he presented several cases of elderly men who experienced improved health after a chimpanzee testicle had been implanted in them. One man stated he felt fifteen years younger following the implant, but didn't specify what aspects of his health had improved. Several days later, at a reception in London, Voronoff told the audience there was no reason why they should not live to be "one hundred forty to one hundred fifty years [old]."[56] He claimed that on his farm, there was a ram that had undergone a testicle implant and was now twenty years old, which he said was comparable to a human age of one hundred forty. At this time, Voronoff was beginning to emphasize longevity instead of just rejuvenation, although rejuvenation may lead to a longer life. He also revealed that he had treated women with gland surgery, although he didn't specify where the gland, presumably the ovary, was implanted. Voronoff observed that French women sought his services because they were interested in "improving their beauty; American and English women [desire] ... that they can hunt, golf, play tennis, and such things again, with all the vitality of youth."[57]

Considering Voronoff's outrageous remark about humans living to be one hundred forty, an assertion with no evidence to support it but tenuous sheep studies, it is not surprising that members of the House of Commons condemned Voronoff's visit.[58] And Voronoff did not escape criticism from the Church of England. The Dean of Westminster Abbey assailed the man "whose theories and schemes are revolting to all pure-minded men and women."[59] The Dean was particularly disturbed by what he termed the "interassociation of apes and man" as a means of extending life. "Where is our sense of holiness?" Clearly, the Dean did not regard a man with a bit of chimp testicle in him as worthy of blessing.

George Bernard Shaw could not help but appreciate the notoriety associated with Voronoff's visit to London. He composed a letter to the editor of the *London Daily News*, written under the name of "Consul Junior," a performing chimpanzee at the London Zoo.[60] The following letter expressed Shaw's view on monkey gland surgery:

> We apes are a patient and kindly race, but this is more than we can stand. Has any ape ever torn the glands from a living man to graft them upon another ape for the sake of a brief and unnatural extension of that ape's life? … Man remains what he has always been; the cruelest of animals. Let him presume no further on his grotesque resemblance to us; he will remain what he is in spite of all of Dr. Voronoff's efforts to make a respectable ape of him.
>
> Yours truly,
> Consul Junior, The Monkey House Regents Park, May 26, 1928

In spite of continued negative publicity, Voronoff maintained a prominent role in the field of rejuvenation and aging. Probably it was his high standing in European science and the certainty with which he presented his results that contributed to his stature. In a 1929 meeting of the Physiology Congress in Boston, Voronoff presented an update of his gland-grafting experience.[61] He maintained that the testicles did not "shrivel and disappear but continue to live." This impression was based on ten years' observation of animals and elderly men. In humans, the positive effects from the surgery included increased muscle strength, improved appetite, better work habits, and a greater capacity for intellectual work. No mention of the dubious animal research. He acknowledged the positive effects from the graft began to wear off after the fifth year. More likely, Voronoff's patients were growing older and experiencing the effects of aging. These were patients in whom he encouraged a repeat testicle graft.

Also on the program at the Physiologic Congress was Dr. Cassimir Funk, who spoke about his efforts to isolate the male hormone.[62] One of the financial supporters of the project was Harold McCormick, the recipient of a testicle transplant performed by Dr. Victor Lespinasse in Chicago about seven years earlier. Apparently, Mr. McCormick was still interested in rejuvenation.

By 1929, Voronoff claimed to have performed 475 testicle grafts.[63] Premature senility was the diagnosis in about half the patients, and added to this group were older men diagnosed as just senile. It wasn't clear just how the two groups differed. Impotence was no longer the main complaint, although, in the senile groups, the term "impaired genital function" was included as an accompanying diagnosis. In diabetics who experienced some degree of impotence, Voronoff used the term "impaired genital capacity." He didn't define how these terms differed.

The improvement in those men experiencing premature senility was reportedly 90 percent, while in those with just senility it was 74 percent. These are astounding success rates. In regard to impaired sexual function, those in whom the problem was attributed to "masturbation, sexual excess in the past, prolonged abstinence, or living in a warm climate" had a success rate of 89 percent. A pharmaceutical company today would be delighted with these results, if they had developed a drug to improve sexual dysfunction. Voronoff observed that in the first few days after the implant, the patient experienced "marked psychic and sexual excitation," followed by a period of the lessening of these effects; then improvement began again some months later.[64] He also noted that improvement was most marked in those patients "who are highly developed intellectually."[65] Perhaps this intellectual group was more convinced of the "science" behind the gland surgery.

In most of his patients, Voronoff regarded their overall health as improved. He described them as having a sense of "well-being," and their typical appearance as more youthful, the "enfeebled body more vigorous, eyes brighter," and the disappearance of wrinkles. All in all, a general rejuvenation had occurred, as Voronoff interpreted it.[66]

In 1930, a writer for the *New York Times* summarized the efforts of Americans to live longer and avoid the perils of old age.[67] These efforts consisted of eating a balanced diet, including fresh fruit and vegetables, and exercising as a means of controlling their weight and toning flabby muscles. And there were still patent medicines, healing mineral waters, and European health resorts available to those hoping for a return to youth and who could afford the travel. The author concluded that old age could either be thought of as a disease "ultimately to be conquered by science," or simply part of life. It was up to the reader as to what "pet formula" he or she would take to beat aging. No mention of Dr. Voronoff's chimpanzee glands, or other glandular therapies available in that era.

Dr. Alexis Carrel, a medical scientist whom Voronoff greatly admired, wrote an article in 1931 in which he pointed out that the process of aging starts in embryonic life and that aging and the passage of time are "inexorable and irreversible."[68] He stated further, "No senescent organism has ever been rejuvenated by the procedures of Steinach [vasectomy] or Voronoff." Assuming Voronoff became aware of Carrel's appraisal of his attempts at rejuvenation, he must have felt a sharp sense of disappointment.

Voronoff's name gradually disappeared from the news. The press must have concluded that, after the accumulating criticisms, there was little of scientific merit in his work. Voronoff did remarry in 1934 to a much younger woman, twenty years old.[69] This did make the news. He was sixty-eight at the time; perhaps he had, in some way, rejuvenated himself.

Despite criticism such as Carrel's, Voronoff still believed there was merit to the rejuvenating power of testicle grafts.[70] At this point, he still looked on decrepit old men as eunuchs and believed his gland surgery would restore youth. In 1939, Voronoff and his wife embarked on a lecture tour in South America to promote his ideas, when the Second World War broke out. On returning to France, they discovered their chateau on French-Italian border had been overrun by the Italians, then part of the Axis. Consequently, the couple fled to Portugal. While in Portugal, Voronoff was invited to give a lecture, in which he stated "old age is normal."[71] Furthermore, he denied ever intending to suppress aging! The onset of the war and the loss of his monkey colony must have induced a sense of reality. Later that year, the Voronoffs sailed for America, where they spent the war years. At the end of hostilities, the couple returned to Paris.

Voronoff died on September 3, 1951, at the age of eighty-five.[72] He had suffered a broken leg during a visit to Switzerland and developed a fatal pulmonary complication. He was buried in the Jewish Cemetery in Nice, under what was termed by the press "a veil of secrecy."[73] The reason for the secrecy was not given. Strangely, his widow did not attend the burial. The *New York Times* credited Voronoff as sincere in his beliefs in his gland surgery, "but few took his claims seriously." The writer must have failed to look back far enough, since considerable material could be found indicating he had been taken seriously, at least by some members of the press and the public.

The *London Times* death notice commented, "He courted publicity and it was with the public rather than his own profession that he was best known."[74]

The Gland Illusion

Did Voronoff become a quack? As scientific opinion grew against him, he might have taken a step back, reviewed his work, sought the opinion of others such as Alexis Carrel, and concluded his results were based on his subjective impressions of photographs taken before and after surgery, and the poorly maintained records of his animal experiments, as pointed out by the British Agricultural Group. He should have obtained second opinions on the biopsies done on animals one to two years after implant. Then he would have been alerted that the implanted glands were mostly scar tissue with surrounding inflammatory cells. Certainly some of Voronoff's patients were enthusiastic about the results from their surgery, but over time, he could have made a studied concession that the favorable results were in the mind of the recipient, and the process of aging was "inexorable." In the end, it was "une grande illusion."

Perhaps the most ardent devotee of Voronoff's experience in gland transplantation was Dr. Max Thorek, in Chicago. Thorek was greatly impressed by Voronoff's early research in animals and the results of surgery in humans. It was Thorek who invited Voronoff to lecture in Chicago and demonstrate his technique for testicle grafting. Thorek must have guessed there was the possibility of surgical failures, although Voronoff was not always forthcoming in revealing failures. Thorek experimented on dogs and concluded that placing the segments of testicle in the scrotum could lead to sloughing of the implant caused by pressure on the scrotum. Instead of copying Voronoff, Thorek devised a technique of placing a testicle beside the kidney.[75] The kidney and fat surrounding it offered a cushion for the testicle. Instead of implanting just segments of the testicle, Thorek chose to implant the entire gland. He made several incisions in the capsule of the testicle to allow blood vessels to enter and nourish the gland, as well as to provide a channel through which the secretion from the testicle would enter the patient's circulation. Thorek referred to his operation as his "lantern" technique.[76] Instead of light emerging from the testicle, it would be the hormone. It reminds one of planting a bulb and waiting for it to sprout. From 1919 to 1923, Thorek performed ninety-seven testicle transplants.[77] The largest group of recipients were those suffering from what Thorek termed "senile atrophy," or simply senility. The majority of these patients were transplanted using simian glands and an astounding 64 percent were reported to be restored to normal or markedly improved.

Only 19 percent were judged as failures. This is a remarkable success rate with elderly men.

But, over time, Thorek seemed to become a bit skeptical about his results. He backed away from the term rejuvenation when he stated, "It is misleading particularly to the laity who gain ... the impression that by certain procedures the old can be made young again." Instead, he suggested the term "Therapeutic Gonadal Implantation," which doesn't imply the specific goal of making a person feel and act younger.[78] Later in his career, he preferred the term "reactivation," which implies that the senescent processes in the body will be lessened and some recovery of normal function will ensue.[79]

In his autobiography published in 1943, Thorek summed up the testicle transplant era by noting the results in the best cases were transient, and acknowledged that "when the fountain of youth within us runs dry, not all that manufacturers sell and nothing the surgeon can transplant, will bring back the magic waters."[80] Thorek had long before given up his monkey colony that he maintained in Chicago, and a pet chimpanzee, a gift from Dr. Voronoff, was donated to the city's Lincoln Park Zoo.[81]

Some mention should also be made of the experience of Mr. Kenneth Walker, who reported his results in testicular grafts before the Royal College of Surgeons in 1924.[82] Previously, Walker had been involved in a blood transfusion project during the First World War. After returning to practice, he became interested in the reports of others concerning testicle grafts. In his address before the college, he recounted the history of organotherapy, the practice of using oral or injectable extracts of animals for rejuvenation. Walker expressed his doubts about the favorable results made by those using these products, claiming that these results were more likely the result of "mental suggestion" rather than a hormonal secretion. Walker reviewed the results of others who had implanted/transplanted testicles and who had reported increased muscular strength, mental abilities, and improved sexual function. He acknowledged that those results could also be attributable to mental suggestion. Hence, he would attempt to be more objective in reporting his results.

After reviewing the reports of surgeons including Lespinasse, Lydston, Morris, and Voronoff, Walker decided on the technique used by Voronoff.[83] This technique consisted of placing segments of testicle inside the lining surrounding the testicle (tunica vaginalis), closing the lining and the overlying scrotal skin. But Walker would not use monkeys. Instead he chose to use human testicles obtained from patients from whom an undescended testicle was removed. These were testicles which had failed to descend properly into the scrotum and usually remained in the groin area. Such testicles are deficient in the sperm-producing cells but retain the interstitial cells which secrete the male hormone. He did not believe the use of animal glands would be as successful as using human glands, although he did acknowledge Voronoff's use of the glands from higher apes had some merit.

Walker reported ten cases. In two men, their testicles had been removed because of tuberculosis. They had noted erectile difficulty and one man wished to get married, which was why he sought Walker's expertise. One of the men, age thirty-nine, underwent a testicle graft and experienced headaches and excessive urinary output following surgery for about a week. This man experienced no improvement from the testicle graft. The other man, who had lost both testicles to tuberculosis, underwent a testicle graft to the scrotum. He experienced only one erection after surgery, which may have been more of a reflex response, rather than the result of a hormonal boost. Walker later concluded the graft should have been placed in the rectus muscle rather than in the scrotum that had contained the diseased testicles.

Another patient was a twenty-nine-year-old man who had lost one testicle and suffered injury to the other during the war. He had noted a loss of libido, impotence, and a sense of fatigue. He experienced a favorable response from the surgery and began to have erections and express a "renewed interest in life."[84]

There were two patients who underwent testicle grafts to accelerate their development. One was fifteen but appeared to be about twelve. The other was a twenty-one-year-old man who appeared to be about ten years old. The fifteen-year-old experienced no improvement during the follow-up period. The twenty-one-year-old man had a history of a brain tumor and had undergone surgery to remove it. Following the testicle grafts to the scrotum, this man experienced his first erection. Unfortunately, during the follow-up period, the brain tumor recurred and the man subsequently died. At autopsy, the grafts showed almost complete degeneration. Rather than be discouraged by this finding, Walker believed the transient positive response served as a reinforcement to continue the testicle-grafting practice.

5. *Dr. Serge Voronoff and Monkey Glands*

Walker achieved what seemed to be a success in a thirty-four-year-old man who complained of poor sexual performance. This man had suffered from mumps orchitis at the age of thirteen, resulting in shrinkage of his testicles. Postoperatively, this patient regained erectile ability and began to experience nocturnal emissions, a sign of improved sexual function. No long-term follow-up was provided by Walker.

Another apparent successful outcome was that of a forty-five-year-old man who complained of "feeble sexual desire" and erectile difficulty. He underwent placement of portions of a testicle in his scrotum and began having erections that became stronger over time. He subsequently moved to Canada so there was no further follow-up.

The remaining patients in Walker's report had illnesses involving the brain.[85] A thirty-year-old man was diagnosed as having dementia praecox, a diagnosis which was frustrating to treat before the development of modern drugs that help control the disease. Following surgery, the man showed no appreciable improvement, a result similar to that of others who tried this approach to treating dementia praecox.

There were two older men who suffered from senility. Both had undergone removal of their prostates. One of the men experienced some overall improvement in his health after the testicle grafting, but this may have been related to improved health after the prostate removal. The other elderly man, described as feeble, showed no improvement from the graft and subsequently died from pulmonary complications.

To Walker's credit, in view of the modest success of the testicle grafting, he never succumbed to the gland craze promoted by the likes of Lydston, Brinkley, and Voronoff.

Was Voronoff correct in his appraisal of eunuchs in Egypt? Possibly they were selected as appearing dull-witted, lacking in courage and enterprise, and suitable for guarding a harem. Eunuchs have been part of various cultures for centuries. Some were used as slaves, others in royal courts as guardians of the rulers' wives. A few became advisors to leaders of a nation. Because they had no offspring, they were not regarded as likely to lead a revolt and establish a new line of rulers. If Voronoff had been a follower of the music scene in Paris, very likely he would have heard certain male singers performing as sopranos or altos in works by Rossini, Bellini, or Donizetti.[86] Certain compositions by Handel, Mozart, and Haydn would also have had male singers performing the high notes. This music would have been performed by the castrati, male singers who, as boys, underwent castration in an effort to preserve their tender, high-pitched voices. For the most part, these were not mentally challenged individuals.

Beginning in the mid-sixteenth century in Italy, boys showing promise singing in a church choir would be singled out as appropriate for castration. The exact circumstances allowing for the procedure were less well-defined, but parents with several sons and experiencing financial hardship or wishing to gain favor with the Church or a political figure would give their consent for castration.[87] The Church did not condone bodily mutilation but considered the procedure a sacred donation to God. The boys would then enter training locally or enter a formal voice program with a recognized singing instructor. Over time the boys/men could remain singing locally in their church choir or advance to performing with recognized choirs and theatrical productions.

The "castrati," as they came to be known, formed a "prominent musical elite" because of their special musical talents and acquired skills in composition and counterpoint.[88] They were consulted in various musical practices and would, in some instances, become "composers, impresarios, chapelmasters, and teachers." Several composers of that era wrote specifically for the castrati, and rulers such as Frederick the Great, Maria Theresa, the French Louis, and Catherine the Great were delighted to have the castrati performing in their respective nations.[89] Some castrati remained as long-term members of a church choir; some became monks, although they could pursue additional activities, such as composing music or becoming an instrument maker.

Over time, women gradually assumed the role of singing in a church choir and, if particularly talented, performed as soloists. Opera music began to include roles for women, sung by women. By the early twentieth century, almost all castrati had passed from the musical scene. There is one account, in 1912, by a Hungarian musicologist who heard two castrati, performing with the Sistine Chapel Choir. His impression is as follows: "I vividly remember their voices because of the shock of hearing grown men singing in the stratosphere, their voices were white, clear, and powerful and had absolutely no resemblance to a woman's voice."[90]

5. Dr. Serge Voronoff and Monkey Glands

The last castrati died in 1922.[91] Because they had no children, they compensated by adopting certain nephews, and extending friendships with "patrons, royals, singers, and writers."[92] The lives of these eunuchs/castrati could hardly be thought of as lacking initiative and accomplishment.

6

Dr. Eugen Steinach and Vasectomy

"Dr. Eugen Steinach, it is announced, is coming to America this winter to explain in person his theory of rejuvenation. New men for old! Within a few months the name of the Professor of Biology at the University of Vienna has become the talk of cities and has penetrated to the furthest hamlets."
—M.B. Levick, *New York Times*, 1923

Professor Eugen Steinach was a well- respected physiologist at the Viennese Academy of Science. In the early twentieth century, he began to focus his research on the action of internal secretions from the sex glands on the development and behavior in mammals. On one occasion, as he examined a specimen from a rat testicle under the microscope, he noted the disruption of the seminiferous tubules and a decrease in the sperm-producing cells (spermatocytes).[1] Coincident with this this observation was the apparent increase in the interstitial cells, which were thought to secrete the male hormone. What was significant about this finding was that the vas deferens had been ligated, thus appearing to trap the sperm within the testicle. The idea then struck him that there might be an increased secretion from the interstitial cells, which might have a rejuvenation effect on the animal. To prove this, Steinach took a group of aging rats, ligated the vas deferens, and observed them for any signs of regaining the appearance and behavior of a younger rat. This rejuvenation would be evidenced by a thicker fur, more attention to females, and fighting for territory in a cage with other male rats. From this experiment, he concluded the older rats did undergo a "reactivation," a term he preferred instead of rejuvenation.[2]

Steinach soon wished to apply this "reactivation" to humans. In Vienna, a urologist, Peter Lichtenstern, had followed Steinach's research and, after meeting him, agreed to participate in a project in which a group of men would undergo vas ligation. A research subject was selected, a coachman who had noted weight loss and muscle weakness, and was observed to have a "scanty beard."[3] Lichtenstern performed a vas ligation on one side only to avoid sterilizing the man, but to theoretically increase the production of the male hormone from the ligated testicle. After three months, the coachman gained weight, acquired a "hale appearance," and a fresh growth of hair (and beard?).

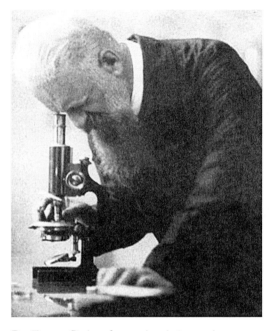

Dr. Eugen Steinach peering into a microscope, perhaps during the time he mistakenly concluded that vasectomy results in the growth of the hormone-secreting (Leydig) cells in the testicle. (From Eugen Steinach, *Sex and Life*, Viking Press, 1940.)

Encouraged by this result, another subject was selected, a sixty-seven-year-old drama critic, who complained of impotence and a loss of stamina. Following a vas ligation, the critic felt "more alive and buoyant."[4]

As knowledge of the "reactivating" vas ligation spread, a surgeon in Madrid suspected the favorable results could be a placebo effect.[5] To prove or disprove Steinach's concept, the surgeon performed a vas ligation on men undergoing an inguinal hernia repair, which exposed the spermatic cord and vas deferens during the repair. However, he did not inform the patient about what he had done. The follow-up on these men was conducted by a community doctor or a parish priest, neither of whom knew the details of the surgery nor had any special training in evaluating the patients postoperatively. Yet word came back to the surgeon that the patients experienced a "complete regeneration of the whole organism—a stronger will to live, marked increase in muscle strength, increased weight and elasticity of [their] skin."[6] If these patients had a symptomatic hernia, assuming they did, which was at least somewhat debilitating, it is not surprising that their health improved after the hernia repair. The best responses were in what the surgeon termed the "presenility group," less so in older men. But a seventy-year-old man who was illiterate started to read after the surgery.[7] It seems highly unlikely that the hernia repair and vas ligation improved the elderly man's cognitive ability. More likely, recovering from the surgery provided him with the time to learn to read. The result of this surgeon's experiment bolstered Steinach's belief in this method of rejuvenation (reactivation). It didn't seem to have occurred to this surgeon to ligate every other patient's vas and see if there were comparable results. If the results were the same, Steinach might have been spared future embarrassment.

Another physician, a Swiss urologist, Paul Niehaus, decided to perform vasectomy on men with prostate enlargement.[8] He based his decision on Steinach's belief that the testicle, in addition to sperm production, also provided a growth factor carried by the vas to the prostate. By interrupting the vas either by ligating it or severing it (vasectomy), the prostate would be deprived of this growth factor and shrink in size. Steinach also concluded that by increasing the number of interstitial cells and production of the male hormone, the hormonal status of a younger man would be achieved and the prostate would assume the size of that of a young man. Niehaus and other urologists in Europe reported success in 80 percent of the men treated by vas occlusion, and that "weakened patients unfit for work become youthful and fresh from the new supply ... of the interstitial gonadal hormones."[9]

Steinach's ideas soon reached Berlin, where Dr. Peter Schmidt performed at least one hundred "Steinach operations."[10] Schmidt's chief indication was senility, but he also performed vas ligation for what he termed "psychic disturbances." In these cases, psychoanalytic treatment plus vasectomy were employed to correct the mental problem.

As favorable reports of vasoligation/vasectomy reached Professor Steinach, he reflected on the success of his discovery: "We may disregard the initial opposition to vasoligature. Reactivation by means of the accumulation of the natural testicular hormone has long since secured itself a place in clinical medicine. And if there is anything that could dislodge it ... it could only be reactivation by means of ... synthetic hormones."[11] There was no reflection on the often subjective appraisal used to evaluate the results. This confidence would be transmitted to others who would employ vas ligation to defy aging.

In New York, Dr. Harry Benjamin became interested in Steinach's research and visited his laboratory in Vienna. Dr. Benjamin came away from his trip with the definite impression that the occlusion of the vas improved the condition of aging rats.[12] Based on what he had observed, he decided to employ vas ligation in aging men seeking a return to youth. By 1922, he had performed vasectomy or vas ligation on twenty-two men.[13] All were reported to be successful to some degree, but there were three "negative cases" awaiting "longer observation," before making a final judgment. Success was graded as "subjectively positive, partially positive, positive (except sexually), perhaps positive, and doubtful," which leads to the conclusion that the overall results were not as favorable as Dr. Benjamin expected. The term "subjectively positive" suggests the results were based on appearance, how the patient felt about his health, or that the patient felt "buoyant." More objective criteria such as muscle strength, weight gain, sharper memory, or improved endurance were omitted.

In addition to vas ligation in men, Dr. Benjamin also treated women seeking rejuvenation, applying radiation to their ovaries. This was a practice advocated by Dr. Steinach. He had exposed the ovaries of young female rats to X-rays and noted what he believed to be hypertrophy of the hormone-producing cells.[14] The idea for this experiment came from Steinach's evaluation of women who had received radiation for uterine tumors or excess uterine bleeding. He concluded these women experienced improvement in their health, not just attributable to the alleviation of the uterine problem, but to the effect of the X-rays on their ovaries. Dr. Benjamin reviewed reports of others who had followed female patients after radiation and concluded that the improvement in these women was so conspicuous that it must be caused, at least in part, by the X-ray treatment—they displayed a "decidedly more youthful appearance."[15] Dr. Benjamin didn't elaborate on how he separated the improvement caused by the X-ray on the uterine abnormality from what he believed to be the effect of the X-rays on the ovary.

Having concluded that X-rays were beneficial to the ovary, Benjamin proceeded to treat six women, who complained of fatigue, decreased mental activity, general stiffness and back pain, hot flashes, and "extreme nervousness."[16] All noted some improvement in their symptoms, although one relapsed after one month. Curiously, Benjamin was somewhat guarded in his conclusions. He advised that a physician should "disregard whatever these patients tell or write of their subjective feelings." However, he seems to have based the treatment of these ladies on their feelings, complaints, and impressions. He claimed his reason for reporting his results was to stimulate interest in "Steinachism," and to promote further interest in this form of therapy. He did not address any possible complications from the X-ray treatment, such as burns to the skin or the lower abdomen, or bowel irritation.

The "poster girl" for ovarian stimulation by X-ray radiation was Gertrude Atherton, a popular novelist at the time. Mrs. Atherton had read a statement in the press by Dr. Benjamin in which he stated, "Women were running to the Steinach clinic from all over Europe … for treatment that might restore their exhausted energies…."[17] She had experienced a decrease in creative energy and was seeking some method of rejuvenation. After meeting Dr. Benjamin in New York, she agreed to submit to several treatments. Afterwards, she slowly regained her creative energy, this time producing a novel, *The Black Oxen*. This story had an autobiographical theme, although Mrs. Atherton denied this.[18] The plot involved a woman who underwent X-ray treatment to make her young and beautiful again. So successful was the treatment that she returned to society and was not recognized by old acquaintances. Her appearance attracted young men, who were smitten by her looks. A number of love affairs ensued. The novel was considered scandalous at the time, and was a great commercial success. Of interest is the fact that the title, *Black Oxen*, was taken from a play by W.B. Yeats, who would have a "Steinach" treatment in the form of a vasectomy to rejuvenate his career. Later in her life, Mrs. Atherton was given hormone injections by Dr. Benjamin, in an effort to impede aging. She even had a sheep ovary implanted by Dr. H. Lyons Hunt, who was better known for implanting testicles in aging men.[19] But over the years, she gradually lost her creative ability along with deteriorating health. She died in 1948, at the age of ninety. Later in Dr. Benjamin's career, when he was asked about rejuvenation, he responded that the most important factor leading to long, active, productive life was heredity.[20]

6. Dr. Eugen Steinach and Vasectomy

The use of vasectomy for rejuvenation was also applied to cancer patients. Dr. Sigmund Freud was an example. In April 1923, Dr. Freud underwent an excisional biopsy of a lesion on the right side of his mouth, which proved to be cancer.[21] Freud had been a heavy cigar smoker, which more than likely caused the malignancy. He subsequently underwent three separate procedures, in an effort to remove all the cancerous tissue. To accelerate the healing process and regain his strength, Freud elected to have a vasectomy. Freud had been impressed with Dr. Steinach's research on rejuvenating laboratory animals and concluded a vasectomy might aid in preventing a recurrence of the cancer. The vas ligation was reported to have been performed on November 17, 1923, by Dr. Victor Blum, a prominent urologist in Vienna.[22] Freud continued to have biopsies and later a course of radiation to the cancer over the next fifteen years. In 1939, after he had fled the Nazi takeover of Austria and moved to London, he again experienced a recurrence of the cancer and was enduring a painful, agonizing life. Finally, on September 22, 1939, he summoned a physician friend, who had agreed to Freud's request to end his life.[23] At 3:00 the next morning, Freud was given two large doses of morphine and died a short time later. Maybe the vasectomy initially helped Freud cope with the disease, but it did nothing to arrest the course of the malignancy.

By 1924, some degree of skepticism was being expressed about glands and rejuvenation. An editorial in the *Journal of the American Medical Association* stated: "Today, no other phase of therapeutics is subject to more abuse and fantastic exploitation.... The hope of restoring youth is such an impelling motive that even the prospect of surgical intervention does not seem to dampen the enthusiasm of those who are willing to grasp at such new suggestions toward accomplishing an invigorating end."[24] The editorial cited a report of Dr. Robert Oslund, at the University of Chicago, whose research showed a lack of change in dog testicles following vasectomy.[25] A colleague of Oslund's, Dr. Carl Moore, had performed vasectomies on sheep and failed to confirm any change similar to what Steinach had reported.[26] Oslund also demonstrated in the rat and guinea pig that when the testicles remain in the abdominal cavity after occluding the vas rather than returning to the scrotum, they undergo atrophy of the sperm-producing cells, and there is an apparent increase in interstitial cells, not unlike what Steinach observed.[27] Very likely, when Steinach or his laboratory assistant removed the testicles for biopsy several weeks after the vas ligation, they failed to document whether the glands were in the abdomen or scrotum. Moore summed up his research on the effect of vasectomy on the testicle when he concluded: "In the many cases of vasectomy performed in our laboratory on guinea pigs, sheep, and rabbits no single case has ever been documented where interstitial cell hypertrophy followed as a result of the operation, and it should be remembered that this is the only morphological basis upon which Steinach's regeneration [concept] rests."[28]

Moore had also disagreed with Steinach's findings in female rats in which the ovaries were removed and testicles transplanted. Steinach had used weight gain in the females as his criterion for judging the effect of the male gland. To test this concept, Moore took a litter of female rats, removed the ovaries, and measured the weight gain as the rats matured. In comparing them with young female rats in which a testicle had been grafted and the ovaries removed, he found no difference.[29] Hence, the absence of the ovary led to increased size. In retrospect, this experiment seems quite obvious in establishing whether the testicle played a role in the animal's weight gain, but in this era, the concept of control subjects was not always critical to the experiment.

The studies of Moore and Oslund did not seem to stifle the idea of the rejuvenating effect of vasectomy. In a report from the First World Sex Congress in 1926, the collective opinion on the question of rejuvenation by surgical means (vasoligature) was "the German theoretical researchers entirely accept the scientific views of Professor Steinach of Vienna, even hailing him as a father of a branch of medicine and biology...."[30] Apparently, the research of Moore and Oslund had not reached Europe, even though it had been published over a year earlier, or because of Professor Steinach's status, it was simply ignored.

The clinical impression of some surgeons continued to support the success of vasectomy in rejuvenation. One author went so far as to speculate that the manufacture of tablets derived from the testicles of animals in which the vas had been ligated might be more powerful than the usual "glandular tablets."[31] What quack wouldn't have wished to obtain such a powerful and lucrative product!

An author of a book on rejuvenation pointed out how Steinach's research had brought notoriety unsought by him and made him a "center of venomous controversy and created enemies where formerly he had only admirers...."[32] The author had visited Steinach's laboratory in Vienna and was impressed by Steinach's professorial long white beard and the clean, efficient appearance of the facilities. He believed one reason for the controversy was the use of the word "rejuvenation" by the press and other interested persons. Steinach preferred the word "reactivation," although to some readers, the meanings were relatively similar. Then too, there was undoubtedly a growing impression that vasectomy done for "reactivation" was ineffective.

But vasoligation or vasectomy did continue to be used to restore youth and creative energy. On April 5, 1934, William Butler Yeats, age sixty-nine, entered the office of Dr. Norman Haire on Harley Street in London.[33] Yeats, an Irish poet, playwright, and Nobel Prize winner in literature, had sensed a decline in the quality of his work. Dr. Haire had become what was termed a sexologist, focusing on birth control and sex education. Yeats had read several sources about Steinach, and Haire was known as a follower of Steinach's ideas about rejuvenation. Hence, Yeats came to believe a vas ligation could restore his creativity and a renewed interest in sex. Consequently, Yeats underwent the vas ligation, and some months later, in a letter to a friend, Olivia Shakespeare, he wrote, "I am marvelously strong, with a sense of the future."[34]

Six months after the rejuvenating procedure by Dr. Haire, Yeats met a young actress, Margot Ruddock, who had sought Yeats's advice about some poetry she had written. A flirtation developed between the two, which seemed to inspire a creative surge associated with "erotic excitement."[35] Yeats's biographer has pointed out that early in Yeats's career, a love affair had inspired some of his best poetry. But the affair with Margot Ruddock did not last long. She suffered from some degree of mental instability, which blunted Yeats's desire to continue the relationship.

In December of that year, Dr. Haire invited Yeats to dine at his home. As a dinner guest, Haire also invited Ethel Mannin, a novelist and "free spirit determined on sexual radicalism."[36] Haire invited her to "dress seductively" so as to evaluate the effect of the "Steinach" operation. After dinner, which lacked alcoholic beverages—Haire was a teetotaler—Yeats and Mannin retreated to her home, where they enjoyed a bottle of burgundy. A relationship was forged, which might have progressed further except for Mannin's left-wing politics and her extensive travel. However, some years later, Mannin described Haire as that "terrible doctor and [Yeats's] operation as a failure."[37]

Despite the romantic interest in Margot Ruddock and Ethel Mannin, which Yeats attributed to the vasectomy, Yeats's health gradually deteriorated. In 1938, he attended the Abbey Theater to see his play *Purgatory*. It was his last trip to the theater, which he had helped found. Seeking a warmer climate, Yeats spent the early winter in Menton, France, where he died on January 28, 1939.[38] Burial was initially in France; then, in 1948, his remains were reinterred in County Sligo, Ireland.

Could the vas occlusion have engendered the last creative years in Yeats's career? Perhaps, but the operation did not translate into physical enhancement of his sexual function. At least, this was Ethel Mannin's conclusion.

In 1940, Steinach published his book *Sex and Life*, in which he laments the evaluation of his work by critics who "exaggerated the facts" and contributed to "popular jests." He wrote: "Those who have followed my work ... will find it difficult to understand that some people regarded my research as directed entirely towards bringing about sexual rejuvenation. If in the course of my studies, the possibility arose of influencing the organism in a manner that would have led to a general regeneration [he avoids the term rejuvenation], then that possibility must be regarded merely as the unsought consequence of the studies [with] no aim other than ... the explanation of natural facts."[39] The phrase "unsought consequence" contradicts the early promotion of vasoligature in Vienna, then Europe and America, as a rejuvenating procedure. Steinach never issued an admonition against the use of vas occlusion for loss of libido or impotence. Also, he might have selected a different title for his book.

Steinach faced competition in the field of rejuvenation, reactivation, or regeneration from Serge Voronoff and his monkey-gland operation. He dismissed Voronoff's procedure by declaring, "It amounts to self-delusion if people seriously believe that transplantation of chimpanzee testicles into human beings can produce anything but rapidly passing effects."[40] It would have been interesting to have heard Steinach and Voronoff on the same panel discussing rejuvenation. No doubt there would have been little about which they could agree.

Steinach was regarded as an outstanding scientist in the early twentieth century. He published a number of papers on the sexual behavior of laboratory animals.[41] He was also one of the first to identify the interstitial cell as a source of the male hormone. Based on his research, he was nominated seven times for the Nobel Prize but never received enough votes to win. Unfortunately, his vasectomy studies were flawed by enthusiastic, poorly documented clinical reports which he believed reinforced his vasectomy conclusions. He never acknowledged the research by Moore and Oslund, which contradicted his notion of the vasectomy's promoting "reactivation" through increased output of the male hormone. Today, the use of testosterone ("T") is advertised in the media as the answer for restoring vigor, enhancing manhood, building muscle, and making the user look and feel twenty years younger. The motivation for rejuvenation hasn't changed much over the years.

Professor Eugen Steinach died in 1944 in Switzerland, where he had been living in exile during World War II. Dr. Harry Benjamin, Steinach's main supporter in America, wrote a letter of praise and remembrance in the *New York Times*, stating: "When Professor Eugen Steinach died recently in Switzerland, at the age of eighty-three, the scientific world lost one of the most courageous and outstanding personalities."[42] Dr. Benjamin recounted Steinach's achievements but didn't mention arguments not settled. He concluded by saying: "It matters little whether Steinach's theories could always be verified or even occasionally they were proved erroneous. He planted new ideas. He had shown new ways. No true scientist can ignore his work." Not ignore it, but learn from mistakes that led to erroneous conclusions.

Dr. Benjamin, at the age of ninety-six, was interviewed by Emily Wortis Leider, the author of a biography of Gertrude Atherton, the recipient of several "rejuvenating" X-ray treatments to her ovaries. When Dr. Benjamin was queried about Dr. Steinach's methods of rejuvenation, he simply replied, "The most important contributor to sustained, productive life was heredity."[43] Apparently, after all these years, Dr. Benjamin had given up on Professor Steinach. Gertrude Atherton lived to be ninety-one, dying from a stroke. There was no mention of her suffering from complications of the X-ray treatments. Perhaps, in some mysterious way, she did derive some creative energy and longevity from the treatments.

7

Dr. John R. Brinkley
and Goat Glands

"You can read whole pages of his 'literature' and not come
on one single statement tainted with the truth."
—Dr. Arthur Cramp, AMA

Dr. and Mrs. Brinkley turned off the county road onto a dirt road leading to Milford, Kansas. It was October 1917, and corn stalks and blue stem grass pasture defined the immediate area. As the community of Milford came into view, Dr. Brinkley sensed the advertisement in the *Kansas City Star* for a doctor in Milford misstated the population. In fact, there had been a printer's error; an extra zero had been added to Milford's population, which, at the time, was two hundred.[1] Brinkley saw a two-story building and assumed this must have been where the previous doctor in Milford had rented office space and started a pharmacy, since it was the only building of any size on the main street. The previous physician had moved to nearby Junction City, a larger community which would provide more patients. The Brinkleys considered turning around, but they were nearly out of money, and despite his wife's tears, Brinkley decided they would settle in Milford, at least for a while.

Dr. Brinkley had left a practice in Fulton, Kansas, when he entered the Army Medical Corps in 1917. However, his stay in the army was brief. He was discharged after only thirty-five days because of "nervous exhaustion."[2] The town of Fulton expected Brinkley to remain in the Army for at least a year or longer, depending on the outcome of the war, and had obtained the services of another physician. Fulton did not have a population large enough to support two doctors, so Brinkley was forced to find another site for his practice.

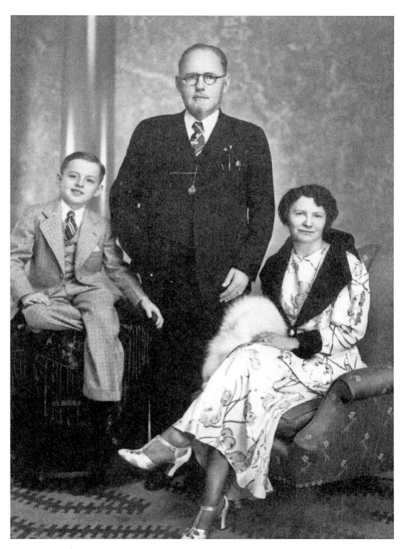

Dr. and Mrs. Brinkley in the 1930s when Brinkley had relocated his hospital to Del Rio, Texas. (Courtesy of the Kansas Historical Society.)

Brinkley's road to Milford had been much longer and more cir-
cuitous than the trip from Fulton to Milford. Brinkley's life began in
Beta, North Carolina, in 1885.[3] He was originally named John Romulus
Brinkley, but when he was baptized, the preacher thought Romulus
was a heathen name and changed it to Richard, his father's middle

name. When John was five, his mother died from tuberculosis, and when he was ten, his father, a so-called mountain doctor, died. Consequently, young Brinkley's care was provided by his Aunt Sally. Schooling for Brinkley was provided in a one-room log cabin, where he continued his education until he was sixteen. After finishing what schooling was available in Beta, he obtained a job as a mail carrier, and while at the train station picking up the mail, he observed the telegraph operator sending and receiving messages. Brinkley believed he could acquire the skill to be a telegrapher and convinced the telegraph operator to teach him.[4] But Brinkley also had another ambition: he dreamed of becoming a doctor like his father.

In 1907, Brinkley married a former high school classmate, Sally Wike, who had often teased him about his threadbare clothes, but who now recognized him as an ambitious, successful telegrapher.[5] Instead of settling down in Beta, the couple joined a traveling "medicine show," hawking patent medicines. In this escapade, Brinkley acquired the ability to motivate the public to purchase a variety of dubious health products.[6] Their travels eventually led to Chicago, where Brinkley, based in part on his "medicine show" experience, decided to seek a medical education at a school which would confer on him a medical degree. At the time, Chicago offered many choices of medical schools, some of which were little more than "diploma mills."[7] As Brinkley evaluated the various schools, he found Bennett Medical College would allow him to attend class during the day and work as a telegrapher at night.[8] The dean of Bennett had once been a telegrapher and admired Brinkley's desire to study medicine. Consequently, Brinkley was accepted and enrolled at Bennett.

The schedule of studying by day and working as a telegrapher at night proved extremely burdensome. There was little time to study, and he was not earning enough money to cover books, tuition, and housing, and Sally Brinkley found their shabby living quarters increasingly unbearable. Desperate for more income, Brinkley began working a double shift at Western Union. After bringing home his first double paycheck, he found his wife and baby daughter had left with the check, leaving him "$1.10 for car fare."[9]

Brinkley finished out the school year, but didn't have enough money to pay for his final year at Bennett, which had become part of Loyola University. Consequently, he inquired in North Carolina, his home state, about becoming what was termed an "undergraduate physician." These were medical students who usually needed one more year of education, but could practice medicine and earn a small income. Details of Brinkley's life are hazy at this time, but he eventually traveled to Memphis, where an associate of Brinkley's, of questionable character, introduced him to Minerva (Minnie) Jones, the daughter of a physician in Memphis. John and Minnie were quickly attracted to each other, and after only a one-week courtship, they were married on August 23, 1913.[10] However, John neglected to tell his bride he was already married.

Brinkley soon realized he would need a doctor of medicine degree to continue to practice. States were beginning to tighten their requirements for a license to practice.[11] He located a medical school in Kansas City, which would accept his course work from Bennett, and enrolled in the school, completing the courses necessary for graduation. At the completion of the school year, the graduating class was driven by bus to Little Rock to take the Arkansas Eclectic Medical Board.[12] Brinkley passed the examination and applied for licenses in Arkansas and the neighboring states by reciprocity. Thus, Brinkley acquired a medical license in Kansas, number 5845.[13]

Brinkley was fortunate to have slipped in through the back door in obtaining his medical license. In 1900, the number of medical schools in the United States had risen to 160.[14] Many of them were of poor quality and were turning out what one observer termed "a vast number of incompetents, large numbers of moral degenerates, [and] a crowd of pure tradesmen."[15] In 1904, the American Medical Association formed a Council on Medical Education and, working with state medical boards, developed a standard of medical education. Subsequently, an extensive review of medical schools was undertaken with funding by the Carnegie Foundation under the direction of Dr. Abraham Flexner. This review resulted in the elimination of a number of inferior schools, so that the number declined from 160 to 85 by 1918, and to 61 by 1933.[16]

State medical boards reflected this improvement in medical education by tightening requirements for a license, although politics at the state government level often delayed license reform. Finally, by 1927, Arkansas was the last state to grant a license through its eclectic medical examiners before this loophole was closed.[17] Increasingly, small towns became the sites in which "irregulars" such as Brinkley would settle.[18] Thus, by a long, serpentine route, John and Minnie arrived in Milford. (One other detail: John finally obtained a divorce from his first wife Sally, and married Minnie again.)

Dr. Brinkley had been in Milford just a few weeks when a farmer came to his newly opened office and asked to have a private talk. Brinkley and the farmer went into an examining room, where the farmer complained of feeling "all in, no pep."[19] He also complained of having a "flat tire," an expression indicating he was impotent. The farmer said other doctors had been of no help to him. Brinkley thought about this complaint, then told the farmer he didn't think he could offer much help, but on further reflection, he reminded the farmer about frisky young male goats. "If you had a pair of young buck glands in you, this might solve the problem."[20] Brinkley may have meant the remark as just speculation, but the farmer, without much hesitation, responded by asking Brinkley to "put 'em in." Brinkley's solution to the farmer's problem might have seemed like overstepping scientific knowledge and medical ethics, but Brinkley had been taught about glands by Dr. Henry Harrower, a faculty member at Bennett. Dr. Harrower later moved to California and became a purveyor of various questionable gland products.[21] In Chicago, Dr. Victor Lespinasse had performed a testicle transplant while Brinkley was a medical student there, and he may have read Lespinasse's report about that case. Lespinasse, and later Frank Lydston, had transplanted human testicles, but to Brinkley, a testicle was a testicle, human or not, and here was the opportunity to put gland therapy into practice.

Brinkley was surprised by the farmer's quick response to his unusual proposal for treating the "flat tire" with a "young buck" gland. He explained to the farmer that the procedure carried a risk, but the farmer was adamant about having the goat testicle transplant. So Brinkley asked the farmer if he had a male goat, which he did. Therefore, arrangements were made to bring the goat to a suitable site where the animal would be relieved of its reproductive glands. Then, under local anesthesia, Brinkley would perform the surgery. This was done in Brinkley's office after hours, and two weeks later, the farmer returned for an examination and brought a check for $150.[22]

The goat testicle transplant must have been a success, because another man who had heard of the procedure consulted Brinkley about a similar problem. News traveled fast in this small community. This man, Mr. Stittsworth, after consulting with Brinkley, also underwent a goat testicle transplant. A month later, Mr. Stittsworth brought his wife to see Brinkley because of an infertility problem. Brinkley reasoned that a goat ovary might be of benefit to her. The details of how a goat ovary was obtained and the surgery performed are not known, but a year later, the couple were the proud parents of a baby boy appropriately named "Billy."[23] When Brinkley was informed that Mrs. Stittsworth had delivered a baby boy, he was said to exclaim, "I've got it! The rejuvenation of man."[24] Billy Stittsworth went on to graduate from Milford High School in 1936, and years later disclosed his father only went to Brinkley because of "prostate trouble" and was talked into the operation.[25] The elder Mr. Stittsworth was interviewed when he was eighty-four and related that "he was proud of what he had done" and the money he had brought to Dr. Brinkley. At one point, Stittsworth and Brinkley toured the country, showing a movie about the goat gland baby.[26] Mr. Stittsworth did not express any criticism about Brinkley's subsequent success and extravagant lifestyle.

Brinkley was well thought of as he established his practice in Milford. It wasn't just the goat gland surgery but his care of patients during the influenza epidemic of 1917–18 that helped establish a favorable reputation.[27] During this time, Brinkley also performed appendectomies, tonsillectomies, and inguinal hernia repairs, sometimes without collecting a fee, if a family was having financial difficulties.[28] When the influenza epidemic subsided, Brinkley thought again about the testicle operation and how he could promote it. Milford was a small community and there were few candidates for his rejuvenating surgery. He decided to place an advertisement in the *Kansas City Star* for an expert in advertising to guide him for procuring more patients. An advertising consultant responded, and after meeting Brinkley and hearing about the goat testicle surgery, he exclaimed, "We've got it…. Dr. Brinkley, you have got a million dollars within your hands and you don't realize it."[29] The advertising man encouraged Brinkley to market his operation as a method of recapturing youth. Such advertising by a doctor was considered unethical in that era, but Brinkley decided to prepare a booklet for physicians about his "youth" operation. He may have submitted an article about his goat-gland surgery to the *Journal of the American Medical Association;* if so, it was rejected.[30] The *Journal* had

published articles by Dr. Lespinasse and Dr. Lydston and may have concluded that Brinkley's use of goat testicles was dangerous and unethical.
At least, Lespinasse and Lydston had used human glands.

Brinkley mailed thousands of brochures to physicians and laymen
in Kansas and surrounding states, enticing them to make use of his
services. To emphasize the importance of his sex gland transplantation,
he had come to believe that the sex gland was the "source of all human
energy."[31] The glandular system, particularly the sex glands, has the
power to "stimulate and dominate the human body and mind." Whether
Brinkley really believed this or not was not so important—it made
good advertising. The AMA code of ethics dating back to the mid-
nineteenth century had prohibited advertising by doctors, but this
didn't stop Brinkley. Fortunately for Brinkley, Milford was near a
Union Pacific Railroad station, and Brinkley provided bus service for
those arriving by train, eager to seek his services. To enhance his practice further, Minnie Brinkley acquired a medical degree from the
Kansas City College of Medicine and Surgery, a diploma factory that
would eventually be closed.[32] She would use the degree to justify her
role in administering anesthetics, a role not without danger to the
patient.

As knowledge of Brinkley's goat-gland surgery spread, he acquired
a "poster boy" in the person of John J. Tobias, the chancellor of the
Chicago Law School. Tobias had become aware of Brinkley's rejuvenating operation and felt he needed some youthful enhancement. Following the surgery, Tobias proclaimed to the *Chicago Tribune*, "I'm
rejuvenated by goat glands." He added, "A general rejuvenation, rebuild-
ing of my nervous system, has resulted from the operation, I am fifteen
or twenty years younger. I don't get as tired as I used to...."[33] Tobias
underwent the testicle transplant at the age of seventy-two and lived
to be eighty-three. Strangely, in 1927, Tobias changed his name to Jean
Joseph DuBois, a name on his maternal side of the family that he
claimed could be traced back to Clovis, King of the Franks.[34] This name
change certainly added another dimension to the spectrum of rejuvenation. Perhaps the "chévre" that provided the glands was of Frankish
ancestry also. Tobias/DuBois died on July 10, 1932, from a stroke. His
death notice in the *Chicago Tribune* was composed of only four lines,
a surprisingly brief notice considering he had once occupied a prominent position in law school education in Chicago.[35] Perhaps whoever

submitted the information for the death notice wanted as little publicity as possible about his rejuvenating experience.

Dr. Brinkley's growing reputation attracted another prominent citizen: Colorado State Senator Wesley Staley. The senator had suffered from "melancholy," a condition dating back at least a decade. In 1922, Staley was brought to Milford and underwent a goat testicle transplant, not without some objection on his part. But after the surgery, he was so pleased with the result that he wrote a testimonial letter to Brinkley stating:

> I wear goat glands and am proud of it. I give full credit to Dr. and Mrs. Brinkley and cheerfully recommend them to the suffering public.
>
> Signed, Wesley Staley[36]

The results from his goat gland surgery were relatively short-lived. Senator Staley died in 1924.

Exactly what Brinkley performed in his goat testicle operation

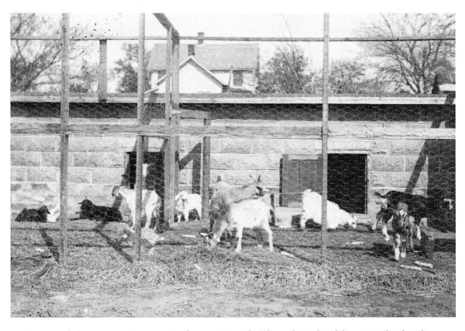

A pen of donor goats soon to be neutered. The white building in the background is the Brinkley Clinic, where the rejuvenating goat testicle surgery was performed. (Courtesy of the Kansas Historical Society.)

changed over time. Initially, he believed that upon being placed within the human body, the goat gland "humanized." That is, the implanted gland did not remain foreign tissue.[37] While there is some evidence the testicle is a privileged site for grafts, Brinkley never presented any microscopic evidence that the implanted testicle survived.[38] At some point, around 1922–3, Brinkley added a bizarre component to his operation. This became known as his "compound operation," as he termed it.[39] This consisted of opening the vas deferens and injecting Mercurochrome into the vas to clear any infection in the testicle and prostate. Instead of closing the vas, he sutured a blood vessel and nerve to the opening; where the nerve and blood vessel originated was never explained. He then performed the insertion of the goat testicle, although it is difficult to determine the exact sequence of these acts. Brinkley believed his new maneuver "energized the testicle" (and presumably the implanted goat testicle). As a titillating warning to the patient, he said, "The Brinkley operation does not confer upon one the license to freely abuse one's powers."[40] In other words, the newly felt libido must be restrained. Brinkley added this hubris about his compound operation: "[It] is the crowning achievement of my career, and if I should accomplish no more than this as a surgeon I shall still feel that I have done some service to humanity, which will live for centuries to come."[41] There is no scientific basis to Brinkley's inflated claim, as would be painfully pointed out to him in the not too distant future.

In the autumn of 1922, Brinkley was invited to Los Angeles by Harry Chandler, the owner of the *Los Angeles Times*. The purpose of the trip was to perform goat gland surgery on two of his editors.[42] Perhaps the experience of Dr. Leo Stanley, at San Quentin, had influenced Chandler to consider this rejuvenating procedure for the editors, but he chose Brinkley because of his self-generated publicity. It is not clear if the editors were in complete agreement with this idea, but they underwent the procedure and returned to work, at least for a while. Brinkley never provided any long-term follow-up on his patients.

One unusual legacy of his trip to Los Angeles was the use of the term "goat gland film."[43] In 1927, the first major motion picture with sound was produced, and it was an instant hit. This left a number of recently produced movies on the shelf, waiting to be released to the public. An attempt was made to graft a soundtrack onto these films so the film could be marketed as a "talkie"; hence, the term "goat gland film." The technique was partially successful, but by the early 1930s, the film industry had adopted sound for their new movies.

While in Los Angeles, Brinkley became aware of the start of a radio station, KHJ. He immediately realized how a radio station would benefit his practice in Milford. No longer would he have to depend on just mailings to reach the ailing public. Brinkley left Los Angeles and began to make plans for his own radio station. Using money from his practice, he purchased equipment for broadcasting and had a building constructed to house the equipment. Obtaining a license from the Federal Radio Commission (FRC) was relatively easy. The commission simply assigned call letters, broadcast band, and power. In September 1923, station KFKB (Kansas First Kansas Best or Kansas Folks Know Best), the "Sunshine Station in the Heart of the Nation," began broadcasting.[44] The station would contribute immensely to Brinkley's practice and ultimately to his eventual downfall. The programming would intersperse live music from local talent, market reports, and Brinkley's counseling about medical subjects. Brinkley would invite listeners to respond to his message, and when they did, they were the targets of subsequent enticements by mail to become patients. Here is one mailing sent to a prospective patient, who had written to Brinkley about his health:

> You have expressed an interest in rejuvenation. I am doing this as well as all manner of surgical operations. I am the originator of "animal to human" surgery and feel my seven year experience entitles me to your serious consideration.
>
> I want you as a patient of mine, if you are considering rejuvenation by the "Old Reliable" method. What is keeping you from me? Be frank and let me know. Your letters are confidential. Appointments when wanted are often difficult to obtain.
>
> Cordially yours, Dr. John R. Brinkley[45]

The radio station offered Brinkley the opportunity to promote his new service to the listening public. In addition to the goat gland surgery, he started a pharmaceutical association.[46] This service depended on Brinkley's reading a letter from a listener and diagnosing the complaint over the radio without ever seeing the writer or reviewing any laboratory work. Brinkley's solution would always be to prescribe a medication from his group of pharmacies. The prescription would be by number, so a person could not obtain the drug from their local pharmacy; only members of his pharmaceutical association, knowing what the number meant, could fill it. The prescriptions were simple remedies such as laxatives or inert substances in pill form. An example of the advice offered by Brinkley is demonstrated in this response offered to a woman whose marriage had not produced any offspring. "Doctors say it is vulgar for me to tell you this ... and we don't think it is obscene [discussing infertility] down here in Milford. What the lady needed [was] Number 80 and 61 and that good old standby of mine, number 67."[47] Number 80 was later found to be a laxative plus an herb, which was supposed to aid liver function. Obviously, neither of these would affect ovarian function nor address any anatomical factors that might affect fertility in a woman. Then too, the problem might be with her husband. At this point in his career, Brinkley had achieved the status of a complete quack.

Many of those listening to KFKB were engaged in farming or ranching. Brinkley would aim his message to farmers by reading a letter from a farmer over the radio, then broadcast a response as follows: "And here is a letter from a tiller of the soil, a farmer who has given of himself without stint, with his simple generosity, that the great cities may live. He complains of his stomach, his kidneys, his headaches, his liver. He writes from Abilene, Kansas—one of my many God-given friends. He must go at once to a drug store or write to the Milford Drug Company and ask for Number One, Number Two, and Number Sixteen. And may the God of Harvests be with you."[48] Note that the number of complaints requires separate prescriptions. If the credulous farmer went to a local pharmacy, the druggist would have no idea what the numbers meant. Hence, they would have to join Brinkley's Pharmacy Association to serve their customers. If a man was interested in goat gland surgery but, for whatever reason, could not make the trip to Milford, an emulsion made from goat testicles to be inserted rectally was available through the mail from Brinkley's pharmacy. The cost was $100. Usually, more than one treatment was required.[49]

The fact that there was no advertising on Brinkley's radio station except for Brinkley's, luring patients to his pharmacy or to the operating room, did not prevent the station from making money. In one of his marketing strategies, he pleaded over the radio: "But my friends, you must help me—remember your letters asking for medical advice must be accompanied by two dollars, which hardly covers the cost of postage, stenographic hire, and the office rent. I am your friend, but even a great baron on Wall Street could not withstand the ruinous cost of helping you unless this small fee accompanies your letter."[50] Of course, the rent was paid to himself, since he built and owned the radio station. The income gained from the letters seeking medical advice, the pharmaceutical association, and the goat gland surgery was estimated to be over a million dollars a year.[51] The income supported an increasingly extravagant lifestyle characterized by expensive automobiles, diamonds, and later an airplane.

Brinkley's radio station provided a variety of programs including live music, farm reports, and Brinkley reading letters and offering medical advice. (See appendices.) A local physician in nearby Junction City acknowledged Brinkley's effectiveness as a radio personality. "His voice was easy to listen to. Its quality was pleasant and his style of delivery was directed in a personal manner to the listener."[52] One of Brinkley's biographers described his radio presentation as follows: "He is a master at reaching the hearts [and] minds of his listeners. In his presentation of facts, no matter on what subject, he is a student of human nature, a psychologist, a master showman."[53]

Some of the conditions which prompted a man to seek Brinkley's advice included impotence, gastrointestinal disorders, psychiatric illness, neurological diseases, hypertension, and diabetes.[54] One example was that of a fifty-one-year-old man who had suffered an injury to his testicles. As a result, his glands had "withered up," resulting in poor erections. After he visited Brinkley's clinic in Milford, a goat gland transplant was performed. Following the surgery, the patient experienced "the desired result."[55] This irritatingly brief summation of the case was typical of Brinkley's reporting. Certainly in the medical profession, only an uncritical mind would accept such a succinct report.

The interest in glands in this era prompted others to take up the practice of gland therapy. By 1924, it was estimated there were about "750 surgeons, mentalists, necromancers, and religious healers offering some form of gland treatment for rejuvenation."[56] Science was thought to offer an avenue to regaining lost years and lost manhood. When diseases were not well understood and there were few pharmacological agents with which to treat them, a credulous public easily fell into the hands of someone like Brinkley.

Brinkley's practice did not escape the attention of the American Medical Association. By 1928, Dr. Morris Fishbein, editor of the *Journal of the American Medical Association,* had enough information on

Brinkley and his practice to label him a "quack."[57] With AMA backing, county medical societies in Kansas that had been after Brinkley began to pressure the Kansas State Board of Medical Registration and Examination to revoke Brinkley's license.[58] They were joined by newspaper owners, who objected to Brinkley's promoting his pharmaceutical association over the radio because the papers no longer received income from patent medicine advertisements. Druggists from around the state also objected to Brinkley's pharmaceutical business, which diverted money away from their businesses. It was estimated that the pharmaceutical association brought Brinkley an estimated $14,000 a week.[59]

In an effort to curb Brinkley's radio broadcasts, the Kansas State Medical Society petitioned the Federal Radio Commission, requesting the termination of Brinkley's radio license.[60] Three charges were brought against Brinkley's radio station. First, it deviated from its assigned wavelength; second, the station was broadcasting what was determined to be obscene messages; and third, his answers to patients' questions were not in the public interest. A hearing was held in Washington, D.C., during which several medical authorities, including Dr. Hugh Young, professor of urology at Johns Hopkins Medical School, testified against Brinkley's practice of prescribing medicine over the radio without ever seeing the patient. He also emphasized the impossibility of the goat testicle operation.[61] On June 13, 1930, the Commission voted to revoke Brinkley's radio license. Brinkley's

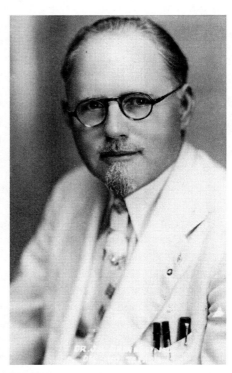

This photograph was probably taken around 1927–8, when Brinkley had achieved success with his goat gland surgery and pharmaceutical association. His glasses and Van Dyke beard gave him a professorial image. (Courtesy of the Kansas Historical Society.)

lawyers promptly filed an appeal, which was later denied. Finally, on February 21, 1931, the Sunshine Station in the Heart of the Nation went off the air.[62]

The hearing as to whether Brinkley's medical license should be revoked finally came about after considerable difficulty convincing the attorney general of the state of Kansas to pursue the issue. One reason for the delay was that the brother-in-law of the attorney general was president of Brinkley's pharmaceutical association. Also, one of Brinkley's attorneys was the son-in-law of Governor Clyde Reed.[63] However, a series of articles in the *Kansas City Star* by an investigative reporter, Alexander B. Macdonald, who revealed some of Brinkley's surgical misadventures, helped force the issue of scheduling a formal hearing about revoking Brinkley's license.[64] Macdonald reported one patient who had undergone a goat testicle transplant and suffered persistent drainage from the incision. After returning home, he noted the skin around the incision began to turn black, a condition known as Fournier's gangrene. This serious condition required a local surgeon to remove the gangrenous skin plus the recently implanted testicle.[65] Fortunately, this man recovered, minus the testicle. Not so fortunate was a man who died after a goat gland operation. This patient was given tetanus antitoxin but eventually died, presumably from tetanus.[66]

Macdonald also reported two patients who had undergone prostate surgery by Brinkley or one of his associates.[67] Both men suffered persistent leakage of urine from the incision. Note that Brinkley never had any formal training in prostate surgery. The failure of the incisions to heal, plus the drainage of urine, prompted the men to seek care in their respective communities. Ultimately, both men underwent surgical exploration of the operative sites, and in both instances, large bladder stones were found and removed, which should have been removed at the time the prostate was removed. The stones were, no doubt, causing blockage to the normal outflow of urine.

The Kansas Bureau of Vital Statistics documented thirty-six death certificates signed by Brinkley from 1918 to 1930.[68] This amounts to three deaths a year over a twelve-year period. Almost all the deaths were related to causes other than the rejuvenation surgery. Recall that Brinkley's clinic treated a variety of illness such as pneumonia, heart failure and heart attacks, in people living in and around Milford. One author has charged that Brinkley ran a "corpse factory," a charge greatly overblown.[69] At one time, Brinkley had been a local coroner, and his name would appear on a death certificate even though he had had no direct involvement with the deceased.

Brinkley's lawyers, knowing information detrimental to Brinkley was in the newspapers, tried to block the hearing about revoking Brinkley's license. A local judge reviewed the issue and determined that the medical board only wished to set a date for the hearing. The lawyers then appealed to the state Supreme Court. There a judge reviewed the matter and issued the following opinion:

> The complaint [of the medical board] was by no means confined to challenge the success of the licensee's goat gland operation, the claimed result of which is that dotards having desire without capability may cause to sorrow as do those without any hope, and the complaint was not that the licensee is a quack of the common vulgar type. Considered as a whole, the complaint is that, being an empiric without moral sense, and having acted according to the standards of an imposter, the licensee has perfected and organized charlatanism until it is capable of preying on human weakness, ignorance and credulity to the extent quite beyond the invention of the humble mountebank....[70]

Needless to say, the appeal was denied.

The hearing as to whether Brinkley's medical license should be revoked was set for July 15, 1930. On that day in the Kansas Hotel in Topeka, Brinkley strode confidently into the room in which the hearing was to be held. He was of medium build, with reddish-brown hair and a short beard. His horn-rimmed glasses gave him a professorial appearance. He took a seat at a table, lit a cigarette and glanced around the room, occasionally stroking his beard.[71] After the board arrived, the meeting began with the charges centering on his practice of prescribing medication over the radio without ever seeing the patient or reviewing any X-rays or laboratory studies. As in the radio license hearing in Washington, medical experts were ready to testify about the danger in this "radio practice," and the impossibility of Brinkley's goat gland operation. But Brinkley was not without his supporters. Outside the hotel they gathered, some to be witnesses and others simply to show support for their goat gland messiah. A reporter attending the hearing described the scene:

> They came like clansmen called from the hills to do battle against a great enemy. They came from all walks of life. A rich oil operator from Texas flew to Kansas to testify for him ... and to say under oath that if he hadn't had Brinkley's goat gland operation and couldn't get it any other way, he would give every cent he possessed

for it because it made a new man out of him. There were butchers and bankers, farmers and railroad men, traveling salesmen and coal miners; the wives of men who had submitted to the operation, there was a regular doctor from Illinois, an irregular practitioner from Missouri—they all came to declare under oath that his operations really produced rejuvenating results.[72]

Brinkley's attorneys produced numerous testimonials favorable to him. When Brinkley was called to testify, he appeared calm, affable, and composed, and sounded articulate.[73] But he couldn't refute the testimony of experts who discredited the testicle surgery. Also, Dr. E.S. Edgerton, president of the Kansas Medical Society, stressed the danger of prescribing drugs without specific knowledge of the patient.[74] After Brinkley and his lawyers had heard all the testimony of medical experts, and knowing this hearing was composed of medical men and not a jury of laymen, Brinkley boldly invited the medical board to visit his facility in Milford and observe a goat testicle operation. He hoped a demonstration of his rejuvenating surgery would influence their decision in his favor. The board pondered this invitation briefly, then decided to accept. Because of the heat in Kansas at this time of year— this was before air conditioning—the visit was not scheduled until September 15, 1930.[75]

The delegation dutifully arrived in Milford on September 15. Dr. Brinkley, wearing surgical attire, greeted them and ushered the group into the Brinkley Hospital, where they were taken to a room where they donned surgical gowns. They could hear the bleating of the donor goat as they moved to another room where an attendant held the frightened kid. Mrs. "Dr." Brinkley appeared and, after a brief introduction, applied Mercurochrome to the young goat's scrotum. She remarked, "You are not used to a woman surgeon, are you?" A reporter at the scene wasn't sure if she was talking to them or the goat.[76] As Mrs. Brinkley made an incision in the goat's scrotum and removed the little testicles, the goat bleated and attempted to kick. The two small testicles were placed on a sterile gauze and given to a nurse, who took them to an operating room where Dr. Brinkley was preparing the patient, a fifty-eight-year-old railroad section hand. The operation consisted of placing the small testicles between the epididymis and the surface of the patient's testicle. It did not appear that Brinkley implanted the goat's testicle within the patient's testicle. The epididymis was then sutured back onto the patient's testicle. Brinkley referred to this as his "two phased operation." The procedure went smoothly and the patient left the operating room without difficulty.[77]

The second patient was a forty-one-year-old mail carrier. Following the injection of the local anesthetic, Brinkley incised the scrotal skin and exposed the testicle and spermatic cord. The patient was noted to be sweating and experiencing considerable pain. This procedure took longer than the first, and on completion, the patient was quite nauseated.[78] Dr. Hassig, chairman of the Kansas Medical Board, recorded that in this procedure, the vas deferens was opened and Mercurochrome was injected. Following this, the epididymis was partially separated from the patient's testicle and the remaining goat testicle inserted in this space. The epididymis was then sutured back onto the patient's testicle.[79] The description did not mention suturing a nerve and blood vessel to the opening of the vas nor to the testicle, as Brinkley had advertised in his recent pamphlets. Also, Brinkley did not provide any history as to what were the men's complaints. Was it impotence, feeling run down, or failing memory?

At the end of the demonstration, Brinkley thanked the delegation for their attendance and offered to treat any of their patients. After a few questions, the delegation returned to Topeka to ponder what they had just witnessed. Two days later, the board voted to revoke Brinkley's license. They noted inadequate preparation of the scrotum of the donor goat by Mrs. Brinkley.[80] The site should have been shaved and washed with surgical soap before the Mercurochrome was applied. The inadequate skin preparation increased the risk of infection. But what would one expect of Mrs. "Dr." Brinkley, whose diploma was purchased from a soon to be defunct medical school in Kansas City?

Brinkley now agonized over what to do next, having lost both his radio revenue and medical license. He might have considered returning to family practice, if he could regain his medical license, but the lure of money was too great. A friend suggested that, since he was still a well-known figure in Kansas, he consider running for governor. If elected, he could appoint his own medical board and regain his license.[81] Brinkley deliberated over this idea, then made the decision to run for governor. He had the advantage of his radio station, which was still in operation, pending an appeal to the FRC. He could broadcast his political message throughout the state. Plus, he had acquired his own airplane, and this would facilitate his travels around the state to gain support. Often, just the sight of an airplane was enough to draw a crowd.[82] At first neither Democrats nor Republicans took his candidacy seriously, but as the crowds attending his speeches grew larger, they began to take notice. Brinkley's platform included free schoolbooks, free medical services for the poor, adequate workman's compensation, opposition to corporate farming, and pensions for the elderly. The latter preceded Social Security, later enacted by the Roosevelt administration. Brinkley's campaign generated some humor, when a newspaper columnist wrote, "Vote for the gland old man ... he keeps an eye out for kids."[83] When Brinkley was giving a speech at a political rally, a heckler kept shouting, "Baa—baa." Brinkley silenced the heckler by responding, "A little louder, please. I might be able to use you."[84]

Some political experts predicted a tight political race, and indeed, Brinkley ran a strong third in an election won by the Democrat, Harry Woodring, by only 251 votes.[85] A recount was considered, but both Democrats and Republicans feared this might produce more votes for Brinkley, even enough to tip the outcome in his favor. As a write-in candidate, Brinkley's name had to be written J.R. Brinkley. John R. Brinkley, John Brinkley, or Doc Brinkley, were not counted.[86] Never mind the intent. Brinkley would run again in 1932 and again come in a strong third, but his interests had shifted to Texas, where he still had a medical license obtained when he passed the Arkansas Eclectic Board.[87]

Brinkley remained in Milford until the first week in October 1933. Associates had kept the clinic functioning up to that time. However, there had been two recent deaths at the Brinkley Hospital, where a "vasectomy" had been performed. The death certificates were signed by W.C. Purviance, one of Brinkley's associates. The cause of death in both men was listed as "encephalitis and meningitis." Autopsies were performed and in neither was encephalitis nor meningitis confirmed.[88] A handwritten note at the end of one of the autopsy reports indicated "Brinkley had purchased tetanus serum [antitoxin] from a drug company in Junction City." Very likely both men died from tetanus, a disease caused by bacteria that affect the neuromuscular system, causing severe muscle spasms. Brinkley and/or his associate used the diagnosis of meningitis, which produces a stiff neck, to cover up the tetanus infection. Recall that when the delegation from the Kansas Medical Board visited Brinkley's hospital, they criticized the poor skin preparation of the donor goat. Finally, the pathologist did not note that a vasectomy had been performed. He did note the presence of "necrotic tubules" on or around the deceased's testicles but could not identify the tissue as coming from a goat. After these two deaths, Brinkley quickly left Milford for Del Rio, Texas, where he was to open a new clinic. Brinkley had been favorably impressed by Del Rio when he was in the army, and the proximity to Mexico offered a new site on which to build a new radio station.

The new clinic was opened on October 7, 1933, exactly sixteen years after John and Minnie arrived in Milford.[89] The devotion of some of Brinkley's employees in Milford was shown by the fact that thirty families followed him to the new Del Rio site. Not all were that devoted to him, but the depression was affecting the nation and Brinkley paid decent wages. Brinkley also had enough funds to start a new radio station across the border in Mexico, where he would be free from the regulations of the Federal Radio Commission. The new station, XER, would be known as the "Sunshine Station Between the Nations."[90] This station became one of a group of stations along the Mexican border known as "border blasters," because of their power to cover much of America. Several country and western singers whose voices were heard over these stations went on to successful careers in radio and motion pictures.[91]

The move to Del Rio marked the end of the goat gland surgery era. More than likely, the complications and recent deaths from the gland surgery dissuaded him from continuing this method of rejuvenation. Instead, he chose vasectomy as his new method of restoring lost manhood, curing prostate trouble, and alleviating other problems associated with aging.[92] In 1923, Brinkley had cited the research of Eugen Steinach, who claimed that occluding the vas produced a growth of hormone-producing cells in the testicle. At the time, Brinkley expressed the opinion that vasectomy produced "uncertain results." It is possible that Brinkley had performed a series of vasectomies and found less than favorable results, as compared with the goat testicle procedure. At least, the goat gland operation paid more. Consequently, in 1934 Brinkley sent a mass mailing to prospective patients informing them that he no longer implanted goat testicles. "No glands of any kind are transplanted into your body. Since animals, many of them are diseased, I consider it unsafe to continue transplantation of glands."[93] If by chance one of Brinkley's former patients received this letter, he must have felt a bit uneasy, even violated, realizing he might have diseased goat testicles in his scrotum.

Brinkley's ability to attract patients to his practice was only temporarily interrupted by his move to Del Rio. His mailings and radio broadcasts continued to be effective in luring men seeking rejuvenation or relief from their prostate trouble. Despite the economic depression, Brinkley's income continued to grow, and he spent lavishly on Cadillacs, an oceangoing yacht, a twin engine airplane, and an eighteen-room mansion. From October 1933 to January 1938, Brinkley's income was estimated to be about twelve million dollars. Most of this income came from vasectomies and prostate surgery, although he did invest in fruit growing and oil leases as well.[94] However, this level of success attracted competitors in and around Del Rio. Seeking to expand his practice, Brinkley decided to move to Little Rock, a much larger city. There he acquired a resort, which he turned into a hospital and clinic. But he never achieved the level of success that he had in Del Rio. The public in Little Rock was more skeptical of Brinkley's claims of success, and surgical complications resulted in five lawsuits totaling $750,000.[95]

The American Medical Association continued to follow Brinkley's practice. In 1938, the medical journal *Hygeia*, published by the AMA, included Brinkley, along with several other medical rogues, in an article entitled "Modern Medical Charlatans."[96] This was not the first time that the AMA labeled Brinkley a quack. When Brinkley became aware of the article, which was often on display in doctors' offices around the country, he decided it was time to sue the AMA and its editor Dr. Morris Fishbein for libel. Because the trial would be held in Del Rio, Brinkley felt confident a jury would be favorable to his cause. He had brought considerable income to Del Rio.

The trial began on March 22, 1938, in the United States District Court in Del Rio.[97] The scene outside the courthouse was different from that in Topeka during Brinkley's hearing about the fate of his medical license. Then, an assortment of goat gland recipients eagerly awaited the appearance of their goat gland wizard. By contrast, in Del Rio, Dr. Brinkley was driven to the courthouse by Minnie Brinkley in their fire-engine red Cadillac. On exiting the car, he was greeted by supportive but sedate well-wishers. Brinkley was well-dressed, and the diamonds on his ring and the stickpin in his tie glistened in the sunlight, enhancing the look of a wealthy doctor.[98] If Brinkley was going to claim financial hardship as the result of being labeled a charlatan, he did not present a very sympathetic figure.

In bringing forward the libel suit, Brinkley and his lawyers should have foreseen the trial would expose his weak medical education and his fragmentary knowledge of why he thought his goat testicle operation was successful. As in the hearing about his license in Kansas, experts were lined up to debunk his practices. One reason Brinkley had assumed a jury in Del Rio would vote in his favor is that he had brought considerable business to the town. His patients would often remain a few days after surgery to shop and see the local sights, perhaps travel over the border to Mexico and visit various shops there. In the winter, Brinkley's radio broadcast would encourage Midwesterners to visit the warm climate of Del Rio and have a check-up at his clinic, where it is likely some condition would be found which required treatment. But the members of the jury were not just local merchants; they were farmers, ranchers, a mechanic, a bookkeeper, a merchant, and a city laborer.[99] Not all these individuals were dependent on the business Brinkley brought to Del Rio. At the beginning of the trial, judge Robert J. McMillan pointed out in the "charge to the court" that "if you find it is true that the plaintiff [Brinkley] is making large sums of money from the public pretending to have medical skill and is preying upon the ignorance of a large number of people, the defendant [Fishbein] would be justified in using strong language in denouncing the plaintiff...."[100]

The trial lasted one week and it took the jury only four hours to come to a verdict in favor of the AMA and Dr. Fishbein. Brinkley and his associates gave weak and wavering testimony throughout the trial, which destroyed their credibility. From this point on, Brinkley's career began to unravel. Legal expenses, malpractice suits, and an Internal Revenue Service claim of $500,000 in back taxes pushed Brinkley into bankruptcy.

In 1941, Brinkley suffered a heart attack and subsequent irregular heartbeat (atrial fibrillation?). During the recovery period, he suffered a blood clot to his left leg requiring a partial amputation. His health continued to deteriorate and he died in a San Antonio hospital on May 26, 1942. The funeral was held in Del Rio, and burial was in Mrs. Brinkley's family plot in Memphis.[101]

7. Dr. John R. Brinkley and Goat Glands

Brinkley's unusual career may be summed up in many ways. One writer described him as "the most bizarre figure to come out of Kansas since Carrie Nation went hatcheting saloons."[102] Another author observed Brinkley's career could have gone in two different directions. He could have followed the course of orthodox medicine and been a "credit to the medical community." But he chose to practice outside the acceptable medical guidelines. Gradually, he became "careless, more flamboyant, more greedy, and more daring until organized medicine caught up with him." In a sense, Brinkley was able to "pull himself up by his bootstraps but never pulled in the right direction."[103]

Perhaps the best summation of Brinkley's practice was an article in the *Kansas City Star* by Alexander B. Macdonald, the newspaper reporter who had followed Brinkley's career in Kansas wrote: "In all the history of quackery, there never was a system so perfectly and smoothly devised to rope in victims as the one Brinkley has developed in Milford. The system begins with his radio [broadcast].... He describes the ailments of men, the systems of lost manhood and the remedy he has in his gland operation.... He invites correspondence through the mails.... Once a person writes to Brinkley, he is doomed from then on to receive a deluge of pamphlets, testimonials and urgings to go to Milford to be examined."[104] Once there, the victim most assuredly would be encouraged to have the rejuvenating operation, provided he had $750.

In a sense, Brinkley was fortunate to have practiced at a time that accepted his bizarre practice. The roaring twenties ushered in a new era in which talk about glands and sex was less constrained, women's hemlines were higher, and the back seat of an automobile facilitated sexual intimacy. Hollywood projected open sexuality before the Hayes Code in 1934, which curtailed some of the more lurid plots. As D'Amilio and Freedman reflected on the twenties: "The new positive value attributed to the erotic ... the pursuit of love, the association of sex and commercial leisure ... the visibility of the erotic in popular culture, the legitimation of female interest in the sexual," all became part of American culture.[105]

Brinkley took advantage of this relatively open sexuality to promote his goat gland surgery. A radio broadcast illustrated his message: "Don't get the impression that women are icebergs and are content with impotent husbands. I know of more families where the devil is to pay in fusses and temperamental sprees all due to the husband not being able to function properly."[106] A man who had brooded over a sexual "let down" might very well have checked his bank account and, if he had $750, taken the next train to Milford. Later, in the 1930s, the interest in the surgical correction of impotence by Brinkley, Voronoff, and to a lesser extent Steinach ceased. Increasing criticism by medical authorities dissuaded physicians from these practices and the public from seeking cures outside acceptable scientific boundaries.

Did Brinkley ever express any doubts or regrets about his practice? He seems to answer that issue in a Christmas letter to his wife dated December 24, 1932. This was after he had lost his medical and radio licenses. He wrote: "I have no idea what the future holds for us. Personally, I would like to discontinue every business that I am in and shake loose of the whole mess and start life over again on a different pathway. However, I have so many obligations to meet that it seem almost a hopeless thought to try to break loose from what I am associated with. There is so much expected from me from so many people."[107] Perhaps the economic depression led to a sense of compassion, as Brinkley realized how many people employed by him would be out of work if he closed his enterprise.

Minnie Brinkley lived until 1980, when she died at the age of eighty-seven. In an interview in 1973, she claimed some goat gland procedures were done in Del Rio, contrary to her husband's claim he had abandoned the operation. The reporter didn't challenge her statement. Minnie's reflection on her husband's career was, "The doctor was forty-five years ahead of his time." She was still a believer.[108]

Brinkley's amazing career can be reviewed by watching a videocassette produced by David Kendall and Ralph Titus.[109] The program originated at television station KTWU in Topeka, Kansas. It provides images and voices of Dr. Brinkley, Mrs. Brinkley and their son Johnny Boy. Brinkley's voice has a pleasant, mellow quality, along with the Carolina drawl. Some of the narration was from sound film taken on a vacation aboard Brinkley's yacht. Toward the end, some years later, Mrs. Brinkley and Johnny Boy, now mature and balding, reflect on Brinkley's career. Johnny Boy sums it up by saying his father was a "medical maverick." Sadly, Johnny Boy never caught on to any occupation for long, despite a Yale education; he took his own life at the age of forty-nine.

7. Dr. John R. Brinkley and Goat Glands

Consider how effective Brinkley would be today, advertising his clinic and goat gland practice. A TV ad might feature a scene of placid Milford, Kansas, and the happy face of a recent goat testicle recipient leaving the hospital. He would offer free transportation from nearby airports. An e-mail ad for his pharmacy would pop up with annoying frequency. But the medical establishment, the AMA in particular, and state licensure regulations would put a stop to his nefarious practices.

8

Quacks

"Quackery and idolatry are all but immortal."
—Oliver Wendell Holmes

John R. Brinkley was officially labeled a quack by Morris Fishbein, editor of the *Journal of the American Medical Association*. Is there a point at which a medical practitioner acquires this label? It may have occurred to the reader that several of the individuals presented thus far seem to be candidates for this designation. But in their era, they believed they were advancing the practice of rejuvenation through the use of the internal secretion from the sex glands. A review of certain literature on the subject of quacks will help in determining if, in fact, they were quacks.

The derivation of the word "quack" dates back to the German /Dutch word "kwaksalver," which referred to an itinerant purveyor of salves used to treat a variety of conditions and complaints.[1] The individual possessed a sharp, piercing, quack-like voice, which could be heard over the din of a busy marketplace. This "quack" enabled a potential customer to locate the voice, then the site of the quacksalver, which was usually a cart or the back of a wagon. The quacksalver was usually an individual entrepreneur, "using self-orchestrated publicity," who traveled from place to place, leaving the town or village before any dissatisfied customers could ask for their money back.[2] By the eighteenth century, the term had been shortened to quack and had acquired a negative connotation. Samuel Johnson, a well-known lexicographer at that time, defined a quack as a "boastful pretender to arts which he does not understand; a vain boastful pretender to physick [medical practice]; an artful tricking practitioner in physick."[3] In the modern era, *Webster's Medical Dictionary* defines a quack as an "ignorant or dishonest practitioner of medicine." *Dorland's Medical Dictionary* defines a quack as "one who fraudulently claims to have ability and experience in the diagnosis and treatment of diseases or the effects to be achieved by treatment." But the definition is more complicated than these straightforward statements. Roy Porter, in the preface of his book *Health for Sale*, stated, "I do not believe historians should start off from a hard and fast, timeless, moralizing definition of a quack."[4] He then devotes several pages to the various nuances of the term quack. In the end, what a quack does is what defines the person.

The medical historian James Harvey Young analyzed some of the characteristics of a quack.[5] He noted the quack uses fear as a motivating force in persuading a potential customer to purchase a product or submit to an essentially worthless treatment. Dr. John Brinkley is an example of a devious practitioner who succeeded in influencing a person worried about his or her health to patronize his drug association. His radio message would prey on a man's mind until he believed he was in desperate need of a goat gland operation.

Quacks promised excellent results; "never a failure" was a favorite expression. Brinkley claimed success in five thousand cases without a failure. Or, if the desired result was not obtained, a "money-back guarantee" was promised.[6]

Quacks were also quite nimble in seizing new trends for their chicanery. The discovery of glands and their secretions opened a rich, new field for quacks in which to operate. The testicle became a treatment for failing memory, constipation, muscle weakness, and failing manhood, whether implanted, injected, or consumed in tablet form.[7] The discovery of hormones became woven into a quack's vocabulary and was meant to impress the unwary that the quack was up to date on medical discoveries.

Another trick used by quacks was to emphasize one cause for a variety of ailments.[8] The health problems associated with aging could be lumped together as one ailment, and a special pill, tonic, or operation would eliminate the problem. Brinkley was adept at claiming his goat gland operation would cure impotence, neurologic diseases, heart trouble, backache, urinary disturbances, constipation, and what else the patient complained of.

A quack's success often depended on the self-limiting aspect of diseases such as a cold or bowel disturbance. If a person was given a particular nostrum such as a glandular elixir, he or she might think the resolution of the problem was due to the quack's remedy, when in fact, the illness had simply run its course. Then there are "psychosomatic" complaints, some of which may have been present for years. The clever charlatan will recommend a treatment which he maintains has never failed.[9] Here the salesmanship of the quack is essential in convincing his client that he will not fail in curing the problem.

Then there is the placebo effect, which has been alluded to in previous chapters and will be discussed in more detail in a following chapter. It will often relieve certain symptoms by mechanisms not yet fully understood.

The use of testimonials is universal among quacks.[10] Endorsement by a celebrity or prominent citizen usually carries more weight than the average person who claims complete relief from a product. One of Brinkley's prominent citizens was the chancellor of a law school in Chicago who rejoiced in the fact that he had goat testicles implanted in him. Athletes are outstanding examples of well-known figures whose endorsements of a product, usually to enhance physical performance, will result in the public's acceptance of a particular drug or device.

Quacks have deflected criticism in several ways. First, the quack may emphasize his methods or pills are so new and sophisticated that the rest of the scientific world doesn't understand his new panacea.[11] As Brinkley claimed with his "compound operation," he promoted it as ahead of its time and his crowning achievement; medical science simply didn't understand it. A charlatan may use the names of Galileo and Darwin to bolster his ideas; both of these scientists had their discoveries and theories discredited, only to be accepted at a later date.[12] The quack may also claim certain religious groups or scientific societies are afraid of their ideas. And there is also a tendency among "pseudoscientists" to regard reputable scientific publications and their editorial staffs as incapable of understanding their futuristic or revolutionary theories. When criticized, quacks may claim freedom of speech or freedom of expression over the airwaves to promote their fraudulent practices.[13] Brinkley finally lost his radio license even though he and his lawyers contested the decision. He claimed he had the right to continue broadcasting his message, even though experts claimed it was fraudulent. But he won in the short term when he moved his radio station to Mexico, away from the regulations of the FRC.

8. Quacks

The ability to adjust quickly to new circumstances is a trait found in successful medical rogues.[14] A totally discredited treatment is quickly shed and a new one promoted. The quack assumes the public has only a short-term memory. As an example, Brinkley was quick to abandon his goat gland practice after losing his medical license in Kansas and adopt vasectomy or a variation of vas occlusion as his new method of rejuvenating the aging male. He had previously disparaged vasectomy as being ineffective, but assumed that prospective patients would not remember or know his earlier criticism.

A quack is adept at making up new words or phrases which sound convincing but have no scientific justification.[15] An example was Brinkley's use of the phrase "compound operation" for his technique in suturing a nerve and blood vessel to an opening in the vas. He never defined where the nerve or blood vessel originated, but his goal was to impress a man seeking rejuvenation. Experts challenged this surgical gimmick, one of several criticisms of Brinkley's practice which contributed to losing his medical license.

Thomas Perls, in a paper on the inappropriate, even dangerous use of human growth hormone in rejuvenation, described a set of characteristics of quacks.[16] Several have already been discussed. One practice was to "pitch" the idea to the media without its being evaluated by the medical establishment. In Brinkley's situation, he used his radio station and the mail to promote his message. Newspapers carried accounts of his early surgical experience and quoted individuals such as Chancellor Tobias, who claimed to be rejuvenated by goat glands. Serge Voronoff used the popular press to promote his monkey gland practice, and by following his career, press stories served to reinforce his method of rejuvenation in the public's mind.

Another trick used by medical irregulars is to alter or distort the use of certain medical treatments.[17] With the discovery of glands and hormones, it was relatively easy to promote the idea that an implanted gland would solve the patient's problem. Initially, the implantation or injection of a sheep thyroid had been effective in treating hypothyroidism. Hence, Brinkley chose the implanted testicle, and rarely the ovary, as the answer to a patient's complaints.

The idea of secret ingredients is one that quacks will use to lure the credulous to purchase their products.[18] They will emphasize that organized medicine has sought to curtail knowledge of the product so that

121

the status quo will be maintained. Or the quack may emphasize that the proper scientific testing of his product was not done, which would have proven its effectiveness. The quack often stresses that his product is "years ahead" of legitimate drugs or procedures currently in use.

Not all attempts at rejuvenation involved glandular treatment by pill or surgical implantation. With the discovery of electricity, quacks developed devices aimed at stimulating "lazy" glands, particularly the testicles. An example is the Senden Electric Belt, worn around the waist and, depending on the model, covering the genital region as well.[19] The belt was designed to stimulate the nerves and muscles to the testicle, with the anticipated increase in hormone production. This is an example of applying the relatively new discovery of electricity to benefit those seeking to reclaim lost manhood. Of course, there was no way of measuring hormonal output in that era, and positive results depended on the user's testimony that the belt really worked. The advertising accompanying this contraption listed a variety of conditions for which the device would bring relief. In addition to improving potency, these included "self-abuse, sexual excess, overwork, rheumatism, weak back, sciatica, constipation, kidney and liver troubles." Here is an example of quacks recommending one treatment as being effective in a variety of medical conditions, not all of which are related.

Because of the unproven statements by the company making the electric belt, the post office issued a fraud order in 1914, which prohibited the company from advertising by mail. In this era, the post office was the one agency with the power to stop false advertising by quacks.[20] Later in Brinkley's career, the post office finally made an attempt to stop his literature from being sent through the mail, but Brinkley's demise eliminated the possibility of a trial.

In reviewing the careers of these doctors discussed in previous chapters, none approached the degree of quackery practiced by Brinkley. He satisfied most, if not all, the above-mentioned criteria for quackery. Brown-Séquard can hardly be considered a quack. He firmly believed he had discovered a method of rejuvenation with the testicular product. Not being able to determine the amount of testicular secretion (testosterone) in his system, he relied on his subjective feelings to evaluate the effectiveness of his "elixir." He published the source and preparation of his product for all to copy, so there was no secret ingredient in his treatment.

8. Quacks

Victor Lespinasse believed in the discovery of glands and internal secretions (hormones). He focused his efforts on correcting the loss of testicular function resulting in impotence and not relieving back pain, rheumatism, liver ailment or constipation. He did not seem to publish any further reports on gland transplanting after the scandalous reports about his treating a prominent citizen in Chicago. He did concede that "autosuggestion" could play a role in the perceived success of the testicle transplants.

Frank Lydston could be thought of as a zealot, a term used by a colleague to describe Lydston's uncontained enthusiasm for testicle implants. Because of his own sense of "buoyancy" following his auto-implantation of a cadaver testicle, he had no doubt that implanting a testicle would have a similar effect on others. He published his results in reputable medical journals and sought publicity for his pioneering efforts. But his use of injections made from various organs on conditions ranging from mental illness to delayed adolescence and other endocrine disorders bordered on quackery. It amounted to little more than haphazard experimentation. To his credit, he did report the failure of this form of organ therapy. He was spared the embarrassment of having his results challenged, when he retired and died a short time later.

Leo Stanley was the only practitioner described in this text who expressed fear that he was in danger of being regarded as a quack. He appealed to his contemporaries to appreciate the science supporting his activities, questionable as it was, in rejuvenating inmates at San Quentin. When he was informed that he would not be on the program of the Los Angeles Medical Society the year following his presentation, he knew he was being regarded with suspicion of being a quack by members of the Society. He did report his results in reputable medical journals for a few years, but gradually withdrew from the gland therapy field. In reviewing the first few years of the journal *Endocrinology*, I found there were numerous abstracts about gland surgery from around the world, a case or two here and there, but gradually these reports became fewer and fewer, then disappeared.

Serge Voronoff began his research in rejuvenation using sheep and goats. He was convinced his testicle grafting increased the size, stature, and longevity of the animals. He then moved on to grafting segments of chimpanzee testicles into humans, hoping to turn back the clock and eliminate the effects of aging. He assumed the evolutionary

The Gland Illusion

closeness of chimpanzees to humans would allow the transplanted glands to survive. Voronoff published his work in several books, and as his fame spread, he became less critical of his work and more dependent on the press to generate publicity about his perceived success. The exposé of his faulty research at the experimental farm in Algeria cast doubt on his entire testicle transplantation experience. He refused to accept the fact that it was a grand illusion. Finally, the onset of World War II and the destruction of his monkey colony ended his work in rejuvenation and longevity. His failure to have an independent pathologist examine the biopsies of the implanted testicles and note the destruction of the glands led to his continuing what amounted to a quack practice.

The followers of Eugen Steinach believed they had discovered the secret of increasing the internal secretion from the interstitial cell of the testicle. They were convinced that from occluding the vas deferens, an increased secretion would result, and an aging man would experience improved sexual function, improved memory, and greater physical strength. Evaluation following the procedure of tying off the vas or severing it was mostly a subjective appreciation by the patient. The research debunking Steinach's conclusions went unnoticed or was ignored by Steinach and his believers.

Not every quack proclaiming a method of rejuvenation in men relied on a pill, elixir, or surgical procedure. The following account of fraud appeared in the *Journal of the American Medical Association*. The article was titled "P. Presto Company, Government Stops Oregon Fraud."[21] The following advertisement appeared in the article: "Men of All Ages—Stop Growing Old. You can recover your youthful vigor and vitality without dangerous drugs and appliances. Our new method tells how." For two dollars, the instructions for the treatment would be sent by mail. The instructions were the following: "So, to build up, to strengthen and increase the blood flow and nerve supply to the testicles, they should be stretched by placing one hand on each side of the scrotum (bag) above the testicles and stretch them ... away from the body, moving the hands from side to side in a swaying motion while pulling. The above treatment frees the blood flow and nerve supply to the testicles...." There must have been enough aggrieved users of this painful, bizarre exercise to have alerted the post office to put a stop to their advertising.

If impotence was a complaint and was assumed to be caused by an enlarged prostate, the following instructions were provided: "First anoint the first [index] finger in Vaseline or mild oil, and inserting the finger in the rectum, manipulate well the prostate gland, which lies in front of the rectum and behind the lower portion of the bladder." How a layman would interpret the word "manipulate" is open to question. Should the anointed finger push on the prostate or attempt to move the prostate from side to side or front to back? No doubt there were recipients of these instructions who were confused as to the location of the prostate and suffered pain as well as dissatisfaction with the results. The proprietor of the P. Presto Company, Edward Lee, was eventually charged with using the mail to defraud the public, brought to trial, convicted, and sentenced to eighteen months in jail.[22]

The above example of quackery was one of hundreds described by Dr. Arthur Cramp in the *Journal of the American Medical Association* and reprinted under the title of *Nostrums and Quackery*, vols. 1, 2 and 3. The editor of the *Journal*, Dr. Morris Fishbein, also published an array of fraudulent medical practices under the title *Fads and Quackery in Healing*.[23] In this publication, Fishbein cited the manufacturers of gland preparations, which were little more than desiccated glandular material sold for the rejuvenation of "senescent, somewhat lewd, and sad old men."[24] The origin of some of these preparations was reflected in the names of the products and the manufacturers; for example, Glandine Laboratories, Glandex Companies, and Glandtone, made by Puritan Laboratories.[25]

Today, the problem of quackery, or an approximation of it remains. Newspapers, radio, television, and the Internet provide a means for reaching millions of citizens. No longer does the purveyor of a health tonic have to depend on the post office to inform and induce a person to use their product. Roughly half of Americans hope to improve their health by taking a variety of supplements including vitamins, weight-reducing pills, herbal preparations, and fish oils.[26] Unfortunately, the Dietary Supplements Health and Education Act allows a variety of foods, minerals, obscure botanicals, magnets, corsets, and bracelets to be marketed for various health conditions with little oversight.[27] Just being "natural" is enough to ensure safety—or is it? The FDA and FTC cannot investigate every person who claims no effect from a product, until a complication such as heart attack, stroke, severe allergic reaction, seizure, or death occurs.[28]

Today, a television infomercial for a particular product often features a suave, middle-aged announcer, male or female, claiming to be a user of the product. He or she will then introduce a satisfied user, often a retired athlete or former movie star. A studio audience made up of varying age groups will applaud each supportive statement about the product. Next, an individual wearing a white coat or surgical scrub suit, perhaps a real doctor, will relate a very positive experience with the product. The cost of the product will not be inexpensive, but if an 800 number is called immediately, a second bottle, tube, or jar will be sent absolutely free. Act now!

While the above scenario might not resemble old-fashioned quackery in all its elements, it contains at least some of the successful characteristics derived from hundreds of years of selling health products aimed at rejuvenation. Very likely, the product is harmless and has little if any pharmacologic effect, except for some "energy" drinks, which might have an alarming amount of caffeine. The positive response of a pink pill marketed for memory, rheumatism, and constipation is most certainly due to the placebo effect.

9

Placebo Effect

"Any mummery will cure if the patient's faith is strong in it."
—Mark Twain[1]

Recall in the first chapter how Brown-Séquard prepared an emulsion of dog and guinea pig testicles and injected this preparation into himself. This injection resulted in a sense of rejuvenation which he claimed produced increased mental energy, greater physical strength, and stamina. He felt twenty years younger, and some scientists who attended the conference at which he reported his results concurred with his conclusions.

In 2002, a group of scientists from Australia reproduced Brown-Séquard's experiment, but without the self-injection.[2] In this experiment, they removed the testicles from five dogs and crushed them in water using a "mortar and pestle," as Brown-Séquard had done. This resulting thick liquid was filtered and the filtrate analyzed to determine the amount of testosterone in the fluid. The result showed an exceedingly small amount of testosterone, an amount far less than what would be required to treat a testosterone deficiency in a man.[3] Therefore, the response Brown-Séquard experienced from the injections was more than likely a placebo effect. He did acknowledge what he termed auto-suggestion might have influenced his response, so he withheld further injections for several weeks and noted a return of his previous complaints associated with aging. Consequently, he resumed the injections of the rejuvenating emulsion, hoping to feel twenty years younger again, as he did with the initial injections. But could there have been an effect from the injections not directly related to the testosterone content? It seems remotely possible that the emulsion contained cellular products, perhaps a protein or fragments of nucleic acid that acted transiently on the pituitary gland to increase luteinizing hormone (LH), a factor that stimulates the interstitial cells in the testicle to secrete testosterone. Without actual measurement of LH or testosterone in the serum, tests not available in Brown-Séquard's time, his response was most likely "autosuggestion," or the placebo effect, as it is now known.[4]

The word placebo is derived from a Latin word meaning "I shall please."[5] Its use in medical terminology appeared in 1785 in *Motherby's New Medical Dictionary*, as a "common place method of medicine."[6] This definition carried further, stating the term meant it was "calculated to amuse for a time," rather than for any specific purpose or disease. In the current era, placebo has been defined as "any therapy prescribed knowingly or unknowingly by a healer, or used by a layman, for its therapeutic effect on a symptom or disease, but [which] actually is ineffective or not specifically effective for the symptoms of the disorder being treated." The placebo response, or effect, is the "nonspecific psychological, or psychophysiological therapeutic effect produced by a placebo, or the effect of spontaneous improvement attributed to the placebo."[7]

What is of interest here is the perceived rejuvenation effect produced by the injection of a testicular emulsion, the implanting of a testicle, the occlusion of the vas deferens, or the radiation of the ovary. The effects include Brown-Séquard feeling twenty years younger, the "buoyancy" described by Frank Lydston, the remission of shoulder pain noted by William Hammond, and the rejuvenated creativity experienced by William Butler Yeats. Several practitioners described the return of sexual function after treating their patients with one of the aforementioned glandular products. Although transient erections are occasionally noted following surgery on the genitalia, circumcision in particular, the erections are not related to any erotic stimulus. The eager anticipation of the result seemed enough to restore sexual function, at least temporarily, in some patients.

Anticipation, expectation, desire, and hope have been recognized by several authors as accounting for the placebo effect.[8] In the early twentieth century, the discovery of the function of glands and their therapeutic potential convinced some physicians and the public that treatment with an internal secretion, for example, the secretion of the testicle, might be effective in rejuvenating the aging male. At the turn of the twentieth century, physicians were beginning to question the use of a "polychromatic assortment of sugar pills" in an attempt to relieve the patient's complaints.[9] Do the pills really work? The application of the internal secretion from the testicle offered a new and exciting method of restoring youth.

In 1946, a conference was held at Cornell University Medical College that addressed the topic of placebos. Among the topics, the importance of the physician was stressed in promoting the placebo effect.[10] The pill or capsule prescribed by the doctor was recognized as a symbol of the doctor, along with his kind words. "You cannot write a prescription without the element of placebo," was a quote from the convention.[11]

In regard to recommending the use of glands, a physician with a pleasing manner would instill confidence in the patient that gland therapy was the right treatment. Such a physician was described by George Bernard Shaw, in the play *The Doctor's Dilemma*.[12] "He has a most musical voice; his speech is a perpetual anthem; and he never tires of the sound of it. He radiates … healing by the mere incompatibility of disease or anxiety with his welcome presence. Even broken bones, it is said, have been shown to unite at the sound of his voice." Not all the practitioners described in earlier chapters were a perfect match for Shaw's description, but all possessed the ability to convey to the patient their ability to rejuvenate. Thus, an aging male, longing to recapture youth, would be primed to expect the desired result from an engaging physician.

The particular method or technique for carrying out a treatment has been shown to have a favorable effect on the result. Surgery seems to promote a meaningful placebo effect, an example being the frequently cited study in which the internal mammary artery was ligated to divert blood to the coronary arteries and reduced the symptoms of chest pain (angina).[13] In this study, the patients either underwent ligation of the artery or a sham operation in which an incision was made and minimal dissection performed. Surprisingly, those in the sham group experienced greater relief from their symptoms.

One explanation for the placebo effect associated with surgery has been the operating suite, with the bright lights, monitoring equipment, the array of instruments, the surgeon and accompanying personnel, all of which serve to inspire confidence that the surgery will produce the desired results.[14] Even a simple procedure such as a vasectomy will require the surgeon to don surgical attire, and the array of instruments will be noticed by the patient before the case is started. Thus, a man seeking rejuvenation by a surgical procedure will more likely praise the result than if he had been given a pill.

Certain medical devices or techniques have come under scrutiny because of the placebo effect, which may give the false impression that a treatment is effective but is no better than a sham procedure. The failure of radiofrequency denervation of the renal artery to lower blood pressure, as compared with sham procedure, saved multiple patients from this technique.[15] The injection of bone cement into a fractured vertebra to relieve pain was no better than a sham procedure.[16] The use of a sham procedure also revealed that fetal-tissue transplants done for Parkinson's disease were no better than a placebo.[17]

In Henry Beecher's classic study of pain relief, he found about 35 percent of patients obtained some pain relief with a placebo.[18] The study has been criticized because the pain might have remitted without any treatment. An example of spontaneous improvement is the treatment of impotence, which the condition might be related to financial problems, a recent death in the family, marital discord, or other reasons which, when resolved, may eliminate the problem, but might lead a research worker testing a new drug to conclude the product is effective. Therefore, any study involving individuals who receive a drug or undergo a procedure should have an untreated group. This will reveal those in whom a spontaneous remission occurs. But not all studies include an untreated group, and investigators try to determine that those being treated have a persistent, well-established problem.

When sildenafil (Viagra) was tested for erectile dysfunction, one study showed 21 percent of men in the placebo group claimed successful intercourse.[19] No doubt, the eager anticipation of the effect of the pill contributed to the success. But there may have been a few who would have experienced improvement with no treatment. Investigators try to make sure the problem is a persistent one and not temporary.

The use of urethral suppositories containing alprostadil for erectile dysfunction revealed 18.6 percent reported successful intercourse.[20] All the research subjects were judged to have an organic cause for their impotence, although some may have had a functional component as well. Very likely, some of the placebo responders were not completely impotent and the hope for a favorable result led to a successful outcome.

9. *Placebo Effect*

Of interest is information provided by AbbVie, maker of Androgel, a preparation containing testosterone, which is applied daily over the upper arms and shoulders.[21] A "multicenter, double-blind, parallel-group, placebo-controlled study" demonstrated that by day 112, 82 percent of the men achieved a serum total testosterone level within the normal range. What was striking was that 37 percent of the placebo group had achieved a rise in their testosterone level to the normal range. Possibly, fluctuations in the testosterone level accounted for the rise detected at a certain point in time. But could the anticipation that their testosterone level might rise have played a role in the elevation? Perhaps Brown-Séquard benefitted from a placebo effect that boosted the "internal secretion" from his testicles, resulting in his feeling of rejuvenation.

The investigation of new drugs has led to attempts at defining so-called placebo responders. Ideally, the ability to determine who might respond to a placebo would aid in determining what the true response was to a new drug or procedure. However, age, sex, intelligence, and suggestibility have not seemed to play a role in who might react to a particular treatment.[22]

The result of a treatment to promote rejuvenation is more diffuse and ill-defined than a treatment aimed solely at a single complaint or condition such as back pain or depression. In a study of the pain-reducing properties of a drug, the research subject does or doesn't experience loss of pain, or at least a significant reduction in pain. But how does a person feel when he senses he is twenty years younger? Is his energy level higher, his memory sharper, his libido stronger, and/or his physical strength greater? All of these feelings are, to a varying degree, what a person might hope to regain. What accounted for the sense of "buoyancy" described by Frank Lydston after implanting a human testicle in himself? Was it a sense of elation, of optimism, or a less depressed feeling about growing older?

Functional neuroimaging has shown that certain areas of the brain are activated by certain sensation, activities, or moods.[23] Neurotransmitters such as dopamine, serotonin, opioids, and encephalin play a role in brain function, and activation of one or more of these has been demonstrated with certain brain responses. One interesting example is the antidepressant fluoxetine, a serotonin reuptake inhibitor that has been shown, in some studies, to produce a similar response in patients receiving the drug or a placebo.[24] Thus, the anticipation of a drug intended to eliminate the symptoms of depression seemed to have been enough to account for the similarity between fluoxetine and placebo, in some patients.

Brown-Séquard was convinced his injection of the testicular emulsion would have a rejuvenating effect. His high expectations very likely influenced his appreciation of what he perceived to be beneficial effects on his body. His health deteriorated over the remaining years of his life, but he might not have lived as long as he did if he hadn't used his "elixir." Without the injections, the symptoms of aging and a sense of depression in combating the aging process might have contributed to an earlier demise.

Victor Lespinasse used the testicle as a transplant to cure impotence. The first patient in whom the procedure was performed had lost both testicles, so to Lespinasse, transplanting a testicle seemed plausible. Although the patient was reported to have regained sexual function, no long-term follow-up was provided after two years. Whether there was or wasn't any lasting effect from the transplant, the procedure probably excited the psychic component of erectile function. Lespinasse conceded that the role of "autosuggestion" may have played a role in the success of the transplant.

Several years later, Lespinasse performed a testicle transplant on a wealthy industrialist. The procedure seemed to excite the man's libido such that he married an opera singer to whom he was attracted. However, the pair separated after several years of marriage. In 1929, the man's name was listed as among those lending financial support to a project seeking to isolate the male hormone.[25] This quest for what would subsequently be identified as testosterone suggests that the testicular graft was not supplying the necessary boost to his sex life—the placebo effect had expired.

G. Frank Lydston was fervent in his belief that he had benefited from the testicle which he had implanted in himself (Chapter 3). The "buoyancy" he described after the procedure reflected a placebo effect. This effect was, in a sense, not unlike the mood elevation noted during the evaluation of antidepressants.[26] Lydston remained a zealot in his belief in the value of the testicle implant, and he continued to describe highly favorable results from the surgery, reflecting on his and his patients' confidence in the operation. He never questioned his fantastic results.

9. Placebo Effect

Dr. Leo Stanley accepted the results of gland surgery published in medical journals by Frank Lydston and made the decision to rejuvenate inmates at San Quentin Prison. He first used testicle implants, then injections of testicular fragments. He did so with the approval of a reform-minded warden and found no shortage of candidates in the prison population. The inmates who volunteered anticipated renewed vigor. It is unlikely they were aware of the new scientific discoveries about glands, but thought they had little to lose. Some prisoners may have been depressed because of their incarceration and were willing to try something new which might improve their health when they were paroled. The majority of those having the testicle procedure were nearing the end of their jail term and this may have played a role in their reporting a favorable response. Also, Dr. Stanley's interest in the prisoners' health must have accentuated a placebo effect from the treatment. However, over time, some degree of skepticism no doubt crept into Stanley's mind, along with the fear of being regarded as a quack, as the articles on use of the testicle for rejuvenation became fewer. The death of his wife produced a temporary interruption in his practice, and when he resumed it, his enthusiasm seemed to wane.

Dr. Serge Voronoff began his research in rejuvenation and longevity by grafting sex glands, both male and female, into sheep and goats (Chapter 5).[27] His early attempts at rejuvenating aging rams resulted in his conclusion that the animals produced more wool and continued to sire offspring. His documentation of these farm animal results was less than precise, and allowed his enthusiasm to overshadow objectivity. Convinced he had made a major contribution to medical science by gland grafting in sheep and goats, he chose to employ his discovery by grafting primate testicles in aging men. His evaluation of biopsies of transplanted testicular tissue led him to believe the glands survived and heightened his enthusiasm for the monkey-to-man grafts. Voronoff's professional and social prominence attracted the press and helped advertise his rejuvenation practice. He had willing and favorable endorsements from his patients, and even humor and satire directed at him did not seem to impair his ability to attract patients. When patients noted decreasing memory, loss of vigor, and sexual lassitude at some point after the transplant, Voronoff encouraged them to have a repeat procedure. Those who were credulous enough and wealthy enough to afford his operation did so.

The Gland Illusion

Professor Eugen Steinach believed he had made an important discovery when he observed what appeared to be a preponderance of hormone-secreting cells in the guinea pig testicle, after vasectomy. Since he was an authoritative figure in science, his "discovery" stimulated physicians to perform vasectomy to rejuvenate aging men. He ignored evidence provided by other scientists, which indicated vasectomy caused no long-term alteration in the structure of the testicle.

One proponent of vasectomy as a rejuvenating treatment was Dr. Norman Haire, who performed a vasectomy on the poet and playwright William Butler Yeats. This simple operation seemed to rejuvenate Yeats's faltering career, as it renewed his creative energy and sparked a romance. The procedure was an example of the confidence instilled by the treatment between doctor and patient. Although Yeats achieved renewed success and became involved in several romances, it was not clear that he enjoyed renewed sexual function. One woman linked romantically with Yeats claimed Haire's operation was not successful, even though he did experience an erotic stimulus from the vasectomy.

No group of men benefitted more from the expectation of a goat testicle than those who sought the services of John R. Brinkley. Through his mailings and radio broadcasts, he conveyed unquestioning belief in his operation as the answer to failing manhood. The crowd that gathered in Topeka, Kansas, in support of Brinkley when he was about to lose his license was testimony to the power of the placebo. When Brinkley left Kansas for Del Rio, Texas, he announced he was no longer transplanting goat testicles. It's not clear if he really lost faith in the operation of if he feared he might lose his license in Texas as well, if he resumed goat gland surgery. Whether he came to realize he was perpetrating a hoax and simply relying on the placebo effect, he never revealed, although in a Christmas letter to his wife and son, he expressed a desire to quit the "business," which he never did. He continued broadcasting his message of hope to those seeking rejuvenation until failing health and death ultimately brought his fraudulent, flamboyant practice to an end. Years later his wife still believed he was a pioneer in gland surgery and transplantation.

For centuries, physicians, medicine men, faith healers, quacks, and others who believed they had a healing gift relied on the placebo effect to reduce suffering. Gradually, scientific discoveries displaced old concepts of disease and paved the way to specific treatments for various ailments. The discovery of internal secretions created a new field of study, endocrinology, but in the dawn of that era, a physician had to rely on clinical impressions and the feelings of the patient to determine the appropriateness and effectiveness of a product or technique. It is not surprising that treatments for various conditions ventured off in different directions, depending on the opinion of the healer. The public, by word of mouth, newspaper reports, and radio announcements, became aware of the discovery of glandular secretions and sought new treatments. Initially, the placebo effect from some of these "cures" resulted in thousands of satisfied users. As mentioned earlier, the men who gathered in Topeka in support of Dr. Brinkley were an example. But by the 1930s, the economic depression and gathering war clouds appeared to dampen the enthusiasm for those seeking youth and longevity.[28] There were very likely an increasing number of patients in whom the placebo effect no longer influenced their health, and who concluded the treatments really didn't do much good. Finally, further advances in the discovery of various hormones, including estrogen and testosterone, extinguished the era of organotherapy.

Today, science education is available on the radio, television, the Internet, and local health care facilities. Those seeking to avoid the problems associated with aging and hoping to somehow rejuvenate themselves are at no loss for information, some of it scientifically based and some of questionable derivation. A glance through a newspaper or magazine, or viewing certain television commercials, reveals advertisements for health food products, exercise devices, healing bracelets and joint supports, all promoting improved health and longevity. There may be some degree of scientific justification for the claims made for these products, but the person promoting the product and claiming to be a satisfied user may been the beneficiary of the placebo effect.

Current research in mind-body relationships may provide a better understanding of why placebos seem to work in certain conditions such as chronic pain.[29] Dietary supplements, certain herbal products, and probiotics may have a definite role to play in stabilizing and maintaining certain conditions.[30] The ultimate role of placebos may be to provide an inexpensive, seemingly effective, and relatively harmless means of relieving certain bothersome symptoms.

10

Estrogen

"Age cannot wither her, nor custom stale
Her infinite variety."
—William Shakespeare

The quest to identify the hormones secreted by the ovary and testicle began in the late nineteenth century and continued into the twentieth century. In regard to the ovary, for centuries it had been recognized that castrating a sow resulted in increased weight and fatness. In camels, castrating the female resulted in increased size and an absence of sexual impulse. Hence, the animal was ideal for carrying loads over a long distance without going into "heat," and was ideal for military caravans.[1] The removal of the ovaries was accomplished by hanging the young animal upside down and making a small incision in the lower abdomen. The weight of the intestines pushed the ovaries into the area of the incision, where they were excised. The incision was then closed.

In the eighteen seventies, Hegar removed the ovaries from one piglet and a single ovary from another. When the sows had grown to maturity, they were butchered and the sow in which both ovaries were removed was found to have marked atrophy of the uterus.[2] This finding indicated that a factor secreted by the ovary was necessary for the growth and development of the uterus.

In 1896, Emil Knauer, in Vienna, reported the results of an experiment in which he removed the ovaries from rabbits and placed pieces of the ovary in the abdomen and within the muscle of the abdominal wall.[3] His results showed the uterus retained its normal size when the grafts survived. This experiment was reminiscent of the research done by Berthold earlier in the century, in which he placed segments of the testicles of roosters in the abdominal cavity and noted the retention of masculine characteristics.

A few years later, Josef Halban performed an experiment similar to Knauer's in which he took infantile female guinea pigs and grafted small pieces of ovary from adult females beneath the skin. The result was the rapid growth of the uteri in the young guinea pigs.[4]

The early discoveries of internal secretions were noted by clinicians. In 1895, Robert Tuttle Morris, encouraged by the reports of thyroid grafting, undertook a series of ovarian transplants.[5] His goal was to maintain menstruation and sexual function in women who had their ovaries removed because of disease or who had "immature ovaries and an infantile uterus." In those with immature ovaries, Morris speculated that grafting healthy ovarian tissue might stimulate the patient's own ovaries to function normally. In 1895, Morris reported his first two cases.[6] The first case was a twenty-year-old woman, who had never menstruated. Morris obtained an ovary from a woman undergoing a pelvic operation. This ovary was grafted onto the recipient's uterus. Two months later, the young lady was reported to have menstruated for the first time, the menstrual period lasting ten days. While it is possible that the uterus may have been stimulated by the implanted ovary, it is not unlikely that the bleeding interpreted by Morris as a menstrual period was the result of sloughing of the implanted ovary.

The second case was that of a twenty-six-year-old woman who had previously suffered from septic tubal disease. On surgical exploration, Morris found the pelvis "filled with dense adhesions," and the ovaries and tubes nearly obliterated. Morris was able to extract a small segment of one of the patient's ovaries and transplant it to the stump of one oviduct. Surprisingly, this woman was reported to have become pregnant one month later, but suffered a miscarriage three months later. Morris later admitted he had only the patient's word about the pregnancy.[7]

In 1902, Morris reported the results of twelve patients with ovarian transplants. In six of these, follow-up was long enough so that Morris could evaluate the results with some degree of certainty. There were three patients who underwent autotransplants and subsequently menstruated for "several years thereafter." Three other women underwent transplants from other female donors and were reported to have regained menstrual function.[8] Later, in 1906, Morris learned that a woman in whom he had performed an ovarian graft had delivered a healthy female infant.[9] This patient had suffered a miscarriage when she was eighteen and had stopped menstruating the following year. The patient had undergone surgical exploration later that year and was found to have ovaries with "many small cysts," which were removed. Morris evaluated the young woman and determined she might benefit from an ovarian transplant in order to restore fertility. The ovarian surgery was subsequently performed, using an ovary from a thirty-three-year-old woman who was undergoing repair of a uterine prolapse. Subsequently, the young lady gave birth to two more children! Needless to say, when Morris reported the results, there was considerable skepticism. Morris conceded there may have been some healthy ovarian tissue remaining after the surgery to remove the cysts. Morris recalled that as an undergraduate student, he had been given the assignment of removing the ovaries from a laboratory dog. After the procedure, the bitch became pregnant again and delivered a litter of fourteen puppies.[10] Morris was quite embarrassed. Years later, the dog died, and at autopsy, ovarian remnants were found in the broad ligament. Morris later adapted a technique of placing ovarian grafts in the broad ligament. After the last report on his ovarian transplant experience, Morris chose to pursue other avenues of investigation. In later years, he made the point that his goal in ovarian transplants was not to make women young forever.[11]

Ovarian transplantation continued to be practiced by a few other surgeons in the early twentieth century. By 1922, Franklin Martin, editor of *Surgery, Gynecology & Obstetrics*, reviewed the experience of various surgeons who had experimented with ovarian transplantation. He came to the following conclusions:

1. Clinically, there is very little to encourage one to believe that transplantation of the ovary as practiced up to the present time has more than speculative value as a surgical procedure.
2. There is some evidence that autotransplants are of some value in deferring the symptoms of menopause and delaying the cessation of menstruation. It is difficult, however, not to attribute some of this evidence ... to unattached ovarian tissue left in situ.
3. There is practically no evidence that homotransplants (from another female) have been successful in the human female.

4. There is no evidence that heterotransplants (from another species) have been successful, where the human female has been the recipient.

5. There is some encouraging evidence recorded in experimental animal surgery that not only autotransplants, but homotransplants and even heterotransplants have been successful and the sexual function of the castrated animal maintained.

6. The technique followed by the various operators on human females, in too many instances, seems unsurgical and too often incompletely and loosely recorded, leaving the impression that the conclusions derived from the work must be unreliable.

7. There is, however, encouraging evidence in all this endeavor to lead one to hope that the subject will be pursued experimentally....[12]

This summation more or less reflected the ovarian transplantation experience up to 1922.

Brown-Séquard had reported little success in treating women with an ovarian extract. But he cited an American woman, Augusta Brown, who had reported success in treating women who suffered from a variety of afflictions including hysteria, uterine problems, and "debility due to age."[13] Dr. George Corner remarked that this woman physician(?) was something of a mystery, not being listed among women practitioners of that time or place. Perhaps she was an "irregular" of the time, not having a formal education in medicine.

In this era, a variety of ovarian extracts came on the market aimed at women with "female problems." These included Ovarine, Ovaridine, Ovogenin, Oophorin, and Biovar, to name a few.[14] A major advance in identifying the actual ovarian secretion came in 1912, when it was determined that the hormone(s) from the ovary were lipid soluble rather than water soluble.[15] In 1912, Dr. Henry Inovesco, a physician in Paris, reported to the Societé de Biologie that a product from the ovary obtained by lipid extraction, when injected into young female rabbits, produced marked growth of their uteri.[16]

Two other investigators, Otfried Felner and Edmund Herrmann, were able to isolate an ovarian secretion, using a lipid extraction method.[17] Both were able to demonstrate growth of the uterus and proliferation of mammary glands in young female rabbits, using the ovarian product. This further substantiated the concept that a secretion from the ovary led to sexual development. In 1921–2, two investigators at Washington University in St. Louis, anatomist Edgar Allen and chemist Edward Doisy, became interested in the female reproductive system. They believed there could be a relationship between the follicle cells of the ovary and the cellular lining of the uterus and vagina.[18] Allen, using fluid from the ovaries of sows, found that injecting the fluid into infant mice and rats produced changes in the vagina and uterus typical of adulthood.[19] With this finding, Doisy focused on attempting to isolate the estrogenic secretion. Subsequently, he became aware of a report from Germany by Selmar Asheim and Bernard Zondek that an estrogenic hormone could be isolated from the urine of pregnant women.[20] By 1929, Doisy managed to isolate crystalline estrogen.

In Germany, in 1929, Adolf Butenant isolated a product which he called estrone, and in 1934 isolated the hormone progesterone.[21] He would win a Nobel Prize for this research. With the discovery of the ovarian hormones, there was no reason to implant segments of the ovary or inject an emulsion of ovarian tissue, nor was there reason to irradiate the ovaries to relieve the symptoms of menopause. Over the next decade, pharmaceutical companies devoted an increasing amount of research to the products of the ovary, estrogen and progesterone. Several forms of estrogenic hormones were developed, including estrone, estradiol, and estriol. Future use of these hormones would be beneficial to some women, contributing to improvement in their lives.

The discovery of estrogen resulted in a treatment for the symptoms of menopause, and, in the 1960s, estrogenic hormones were used for birth control. Menopause itself underwent a change in concept. No longer was it regarded as part of a woman's life as she entered her forties, but as a pathologic condition which could be treated. The term "medicalization" has been applied to a condition which is part of normal aging in a woman.[22] After the discovery of estrogen, and for the next few decades, the hormone was used to relieve the symptoms of menopause, then discontinued when it was thought the symptoms were relieved and the hormone could safely be withdrawn.

During the 1950s, a number of investigators, including Dr. William Masters (of Masters and Johnson sex research fame), began to consider the effect of estrogen therapy in older women. Masters came to believe his research justified the continuation of estrogen therapy into a woman's later years.[23] He believed the women he studied led more active and meaningful lives. This idea of rejuvenating older women became part of a growing interest in long-term estrogen treatment. Gradually, physicians began to accept the continued use of hormones after menopause. Some vociferous spokesmen began to sell the idea of estrogen for life.[24] Following a series of international meetings on aging and menopause, the opinion emerged that more frequent use of estrogen was indicated in the health care of post-menopausal women.[25]

But problems with long-term estrogen replacement began to emerge. The incidence of uterine endometrial cancer began to rise.[26] There were also reports of increased breast cancer in estrogen users.[27] To reduce the incidence of uterine cancer, a low dose of progesterone was added to the hormone replacement regimen. This addition of progesterone negated the over-stimulation of the uterine lining by estrogen alone.

Although the use of female hormone replacement was thought to have a beneficial effect on the cardiovascular system, later reports indicated there could be risks.[28] However, another report indicated there were no long-term risks to the cardiovascular system in women taking hormone replacement.[29] Such conflicting reports only raised alarm and confusion in women of menopausal age and their physicians. Over the past thirty years, the use of hormone replacement therapy in menopausal women increased, then declined as the fear of uterine cancer, breast cancer and circulatory ailments tempered the enthusiasm for taking hormones.[30] The most common indication for hormone treatment is vasomotor instability ("hot flashes").[31] Approximately 30 percent of postmenopausal women have osteoporosis, and this is another indication for hormone replacement therapy.[32] Other benefits include reversing atrophic vaginitis and preventing urinary tract infections.[33] Cognitive benefits are controversial; there is no definite indication that hormone replacement will reduce the risk of Alzheimer's Disease.[34]

The results of the Women's Health Initiative showed that breast cancer, non-fatal heart disease, stroke, and pulmonary embolism are increased with hormone treatment.[35] But it is possible that the apparent increase in breast cancer reflects greater concern for the disease, leading to earlier detection. There are other means of preventing osteoporosis rather than hormones; increased calcium and vitamin D intake are also effective, as is increased exercise.[36] It would seem that the use of hormones in menopausal women to relieve symptoms of menopause is reasonable, but the long-term use as a means of avoiding aging or seeking rejuvenation could lead to certain damaging health problems.

A relatively recent report on the effect of estradiol on the cardiovascular system found that the changes in the carotid artery were less in women who started on estrogen within six years after menopause, as compared with those who were started on estrogen ten years or longer after menopause.[37] However, the study was not powered to determine if the incidence of coronary artery disease was lessened, and "extrapolation of these results to clinical events would be premature."

As the mystery of hormone production from the ovaries was solved, it was found that estrogen produced maturation of the ovum, and that progesterone, which is produced by the corpus luteum after the ovum has been released, prepares the uterus for fertilization. If fertilization has not occurred, the secretion of progesterone decreases and after a few days ceases. The lining of the uterus is shed and menstruation occurs.[38] The cycle is repeated as stimulation of the ovary from the pituitary gland brings about maturation of another ovum.

The story of how women's hormones became used for contraception probably began in 1919, when Ludwig Haberlandt performed an experiment in which the ovaries from a pregnant rabbit were implanted into a non-pregnant female caged with male rabbits. Despite frequent coitus, the female remained infertile. Haberlandt recognized that the corpus luteum from the implanted ovaries was responsible. By 1931, Haberlandt forecast the use of a contraceptive agent that would inhibit ovulation and become a method of choice in birth control.[39]

Following up on this idea, three investigators at the University of Pennsylvania reported that injections of the recently discovered hormone progesterone, the secretion from the corpus luteum, prevented ovulation in rabbits.[40] Despite the fact that the hormone secreted by the corpus luteum prevented ovulation, there were no immediate steps taken to promote this finding as a commercial venture for clinical use. However, the publication by the group at the University of Pennsylvania attracted the attention of Gregory Goodwin Pincus and M.C. Chang. Pincus had been on Harvard's faculty, but had been let go because of personality problems and a tendency to report his work to the press.[41] Pincus subsequently found work at Clark University in Wooster,

Massachusetts. There he, along with a colleague, Hudson Hoagland, founded the Wooster Foundation for Experimental Biology. At Wooster, he could pursue the idea of discovering a product that would prevent conception.[42] Interest in limiting the size of a family goes back centuries. In the early twentieth century, pregnancy could be prevented by a man using a condom or a woman using a diaphragm and spermicidal jelly. The rhythm method had also become a means of birth control, as knowledge of the physiology of ovulation became known. Abortion remained an option, if all the above failed.

A leading proponent of what became known as the Planned Parenthood Federation of America was Margaret Sanger. She was born Margaret Higgins in 1897 into a Catholic family that eventually reached a total of eleven children. Early in her life, she sensed that eleven children were too many, and were a contributing factor to her mother's death at the age of fifty.[43] As a young woman, she studied nursing, and in 1916 opened a birth control clinic in Brooklyn. At a hospital dance she met and later married William Sanger, a painter and architect. The couple had three children. But Margaret Sanger did not relish the role of mother and homemaker.[44] She recognized the plight of women who were trapped in a marriage where five, six, or more children would slowly erode a woman's health. She later divorced her husband and devoted her efforts to birth control. Some years later, she met Gregory Pincus to discuss his research and expound on the need for a pill that would inhibit fertility.

Another woman would play an important role in the research and development of a birth control pill; this was Katherine McCormick.[45] She had married Stanley McCormick, son of Cyrus McCormick, founder of International Harvester, and the brother of Harold McCormick, who had undergone a testicle transplant by Dr. Lespinasse (Chapter 2). Stanley developed schizophrenia during the early months of their marriage, and Katherine and the McCormick family provided care for Stanley during the remaining years of his life. Katherine had become interested in women's rights, and following the ratification of the Nineteenth Amendment, she turned her attention to population control and the birth control movement.[46] Following the death of her husband and the settlement of his sizable estate, Katherine possessed a sizable fortune and was able to support efforts directed at the development of a contraceptive pill.

The Gland Illusion

The Second World War interrupted Pincus's research, but following the war, he resumed research on progesterone as an agent for inhibiting ovulation. Katherine McCormick subsequently became a financial backer of Pincus, and with her background as an MIT graduate in science, she understood the importance of Pincus's approach. Although Pincus had shown he could inhibit ovulation in rabbits using progesterone, he would need to test the effectiveness of this concept in humans. Following a meeting with Margaret Sanger in 1950, Pincus began to formulate a plan for testing progesterone as a birth control drug.[47] He would need a physician who practiced gynecology and obstetrics and was recognized as an expert in infertility and reproduction. Such a person was Dr. John Rock, who had previously had contact with Pincus when he was an assistant in Pincus's laboratory studying in vitro fertilization.[48] Rock was a Catholic and had set up a clinic for advising women on the rhythm method for avoiding pregnancy. Rock had numerous women in his clinic who were hoping for an effective method to avoid having more children. Rock was limited by Massachusetts law prohibiting the advertisement of birth control, and by the Catholic Church. In his clinic, he also encountered women who had been unable to conceive, and he began to consider the use of hormones to overcome infertility. Pincus had suggested to Rock that he try various combinations of estrogen and progesterone on the infertile women. Consequently, Rock treated a group of infertile women with estrogen and progesterone, and some did become pregnant, but some women stopped menstruating. This offered a clue that the hormones might inhibit ovulation.

In 1954, Pincus obtained financial support from Planned Parenthood and obtained two synthetic progestins, one from Searle in the U.S., and the other from Syntex, a company recently formed in Mexico.[49] Back in the 1940s, a chemist, Russell Marker, had been searching for an inexpensive source of progesterone. He became aware of a yam grown in Mexico from which progesterone could be extracted. Marker subsequently formed the company Syntex. Later Carl Djerassi would take up the work on progesterone and ultimately develop a synthetic progestin termed norethindrone.[50] At Searle, Frank Colton synthesized the progestin named norethyndrel. In 1953, Pincus and Chang tested both products and chose Searle's, although the two were almost identical in their hormonal effects.[51] Both synthetic progestins were effective when taken orally. The initial trial of a pill, later named Enovid, was to be on infertile women, with the idea of starting them on the pill and then withdrawing it to see if a normal menstrual cycle would ensue. When an application was made to the FDA, the pill was approved for menstrual irregularities in 1957, but to use the pill as a contraceptive would require further evaluation.[52]

But where would Pincus and Rock turn to seek patients on whom to test the contraceptive properties of the progestins? Pincus had lectured in Puerto Rico and had been impressed with health care on the island. Birth control had been legal in Puerto Rico since 1957.[53] The island had a relatively high birth rate and a dense population for its size. Women often sought surgical sterilization after multiple births because it was an effective means of birth control. In a sense, for women in Puerto Rico to be able to take a pill on a daily basis as a contraceptive would have a rejuvenating effect on their lives.

By 1956, Pincus was ready to test the new synthetic progesterone on Puerto Rican women. With the help of local physicians, 221 women were enrolled in the study.[54] There were reports of some women experiencing nausea, breast pain, headaches, and abdominal pain, but these complaints were not frequent enough to stop the study. John Rock had used the drug on his patients for menstrual problems and infertility and had not observed any harmful effects. As noted earlier, he had treated a group of infertile women with an estrogen-progesterone combination and had some success in producing a pregnancy. He had noted that women stopped menstruating on this hormonal combination, some thinking they were pregnant. This offered a further clue that the hormones would inhibit the menstrual cycle.

The pill had been approved by the FDA for use in menstrual disorders, and the Searle Company assumed that an application for its use as a contraceptive would speed through the approval process. However, because there was no long-term evaluation of the women who had taken Enovid, as the pill was called, the FDA took its time on the evaluation. Was there a risk of cancer, cardiovascular disease, or gastrointestinal disorders? These questions would need to be addressed before the application was approved. The FDA conducted interviews from around the U.S. with doctors who had some experience with prescribing Enovid and could provide some guidance as to what risks there might be in its long-term use as a contraceptive. One physician who raised concerns about Enovid as a contraceptive was Dr. Edward Tyler, head of a Planned Parenthood clinic in Los Angeles.[55] Some of his patients had experienced abnormal bleeding, weight gain, and fluid retention while on the drug. The FDA considered Tyler a neutral observer because he had no financial interest in Enovid. Finally, after reviewing the responses of other physicians who had reported their experience with Enovid, Dr. Tyler weighed the use of diaphragms and condoms versus the risks that pregnancy carried with it and gave his approval for the pill.[56] After evaluating the various issues surrounding Enovid as a contraceptive, the FDA granted approval on May 9, 1960, and on June 23 approved the 10 milligram dose.[57] The pill was no longer a dream of Margaret Sanger and Katherine McCormick, nor an illusion in the minds of some skeptics.

Gradually, state laws prohibiting the sale, distribution and advertisement of birth control methods, including the pill, were rescinded. Today approximately twelve million women in the United States take the pill.[58] During the first decade of its use, the occurrence of blood clots became a concern, but gradually the dose of hormones in the pill was reduced so there is only a fraction of the amount that was in the original preparation.[59]

Did the pill bring about a sexual revolution? Probably the short skirts of the 1920s and the invention of the automobile, a couch on wheels, contributed as much or more than the pill. Alfred Kinsey's study of sexual behavior in 1947 indicated that 85 percent of white men had engaged in premarital sex.[60] Presumably the vast majority of these encounters involved women. So to say that the pill encouraged promiscuity is ignoring the sexual behavior earlier in the twentieth century. It should be remembered that the pill played a role in freeing women from an unwanted pregnancy, provided an opportunity for an education, and encouraged "meaningful employment."[61]

11

Testosterone

"I realize you are anxious to build up great strength and power as soon as possible."
—Charles Atlas, Dynamic Tension System

The quest to identify the internal secretion from the testicle that produced a masculine body and behavior gained momentum in the 1920s. Scientists were highly skeptical of the testicle transplant reports of success and the boastful claims of makers of pills and capsules derived from testicular material. The gland illusion, based on the practices described earlier in this text, was about to be swept away.

In 1929, T.F. Gallagher and Fred Koch, at the University of Chicago, isolated a product from the lipid fraction of bulls' testicles which, when injected into capons, restored their virility.[1] This product was then administered to an eunuchoid man and, after a series of injections, the man experienced the onset of sexual desire and erectile function. However, after a series of injections, the supply of hormone extracted from the bulls' testicles was exhausted and the man lapsed into his previous eunuchoid condition. These two investigators chose not to name the secretion until it could be identified chemically.

In 1935, Ernest Laquer, from the Organon Company in the Netherlands, also isolated a product from bulls' testicles, which he named testosterone.[2] At about the same time, Adolf Butenandt, who had previously discovered estrone, isolated a product from human male urine, which he named androsterone. Subsequently, Butenandt and a Swiss chemist, Leopold Ruzika, found that testosterone could be synthesized from cholesterol, thus eliminating the tedious process of extracting testosterone from bulls' testicles or urine. The 1939 Nobel Prize in chemistry was awarded to Butenandt and Ruzika for their discoveries.[3]

147

The Gland Illusion

At this time, the commercial preparation of testosterone in the form of testosterone propionate commenced.

But the preparation of testosterone did not prove to be an immediate bonanza for the pharmaceutical companies. Had the hormone been available in the "roaring twenties," the use of testosterone might have met with more enthusiasm. However, the economic depression and subsequent onset of World War II seemed to dampen interest in the hormone. One explanation as to why testosterone did not become more widely used was that there was a "sexual conservatism" at the time during which a man and woman married, produced children, and the wife then experienced menopause.[4] There seemed little need to consider testosterone as a sexual stimulant in the couple's middle age. The symptoms of decreased strength, decreased libido and erectile ability, the increase in abdominal fat, and wavering memory were thought to be part of aging. Years later these symptoms would be thought of as treatable with the male hormone.

In 1951, there was a favorable report on the use of testosterone in older men complaining of the symptoms of aging. The results showed improvement in a "sense of well-being, improved physical strength, and greater sexual activity."[5] A somewhat contrary report that year addressed the "widespread problem of early impotence in the male."[6] The author believed that "sexual enjoyment of aging persons will be increased and stabilized when the distorted ideals of what constitute sexual attractiveness are replaced with an affectionate and dignified personal relationship." If strong morning erections occurred in older men, then psychotherapy might be effective, if sexual relations were unsatisfactory. Clearly, such men were not completely impotent. The author added, "The use of testosterone has been outrageously exploited." This statement seems to imply that the author had evaluated older men in whom testosterone had not been successful in restoring sexual function.

One of the risks of testosterone therapy has been the occurrence of prostate cancer. In 1955, an article indicated that the use of testosterone in older men did not cause cancer.[7] Testosterone propionate was administered to one hundred men for up to five years and only one case of prostate cancer was detected. This was in an eighty-year-old man evaluated seven years after the testosterone study had ended. The authors concluded testosterone treatment did not cause or activate prostate cancer. However, this was in an era before prostate specific antigen (PSA) testing was available. There might have been other men in whom prostate cancer was present, but it did not present clinically during the course of the study. Also of interest in the report was the finding that during the period covered by this study, prostate enlargement occurred in twenty-seven men in the testosterone group and thirty-four in the control group. This indicates that testosterone treatment did not invariably lead to prostate enlargement.

By 1992, when PSA testing became available, one report showed when testosterone injections were given to older men with low testosterone, the PSA level rose slightly, but there was no change in the size of the prostate.[8] The men reported an increase in libido and a sense of well-being. This study did not address the issue of prostate cancer.

In 2005, an extended review article addressed the issues of androgen (testosterone) replacement in the aging male.[9] The authors point out in the year 2000, there were 14,452,000 men over the age of sixty-five. By the year 2030, the number was expected to rise to 31,343,000. Approximately 30 percent of men age sixty to seventy have low testosterone, and the number rises to 70 percent in the age group seventy to eighty. Hence, there is an increasing potential market for testosterone replacement therapy. However, it can be difficult to separate the symptoms of aging such as loss of energy, depressed mood, memory problems, and decreased physical strength from the symptoms of testosterone deficiency. By the time a man has reached eighty, it is estimated he has lost about 35 percent of his muscle mass, which explains the loss of physical strength. Some of the above mentioned symptoms have been known to respond to testosterone treatment. It has been known for years that testosterone builds muscle.[10] In regard to cognition, a report of 407 men followed for up to ten years showed those with higher testosterone levels scored higher in "visual and verbal memory, visiospacial functioning, and visiomotor scanning."[11] However, the authors of this study noted the results from five other placebo-controlled studies on cognitive function showed mixed results.

One of the difficulties in identifying the symptoms of low testosterone, sometimes referred to as hypogonadism, in older men is determining which symptoms are most indicative of testosterone deficiency. In a 2007 article, the conclusion was reached that the indications for treatment were not yet well defined.[12] Certainly not every elderly male noting occasional memory lapse, some degree of fatigue, or decreased strength requires testosterone therapy, unless the symptoms are particularly bothersome and laboratory tests show a low testosterone. Testosterone treatment has been shown to improve sexual dysfunction.[13] However, a review of other clinical trials revealed inconsistent results. Research has shown that testosterone increases penile nitric oxide, which produces relaxation of the corpus cavernosus smooth muscle of the penis, resulting in an erection.[14] However, vascular disease and/or neuropathy may impair the mechanism of erection, and testosterone treatment may have little effect on erectile ability.

Adverse effects have been reported in men receiving testosterone. In a group of 209 men, twenty-nine reported a variety of problems.[15] Of particular interest was the occurrence of cardiovascular events in twenty-three men receiving testosterone compared with five men in the placebo group. Ten men suffered specific heart-related adverse events compared with only one in the placebo group. It should be noted that 85 percent of the men in the testosterone group had a history of hypertension, a finding not unexpected in this age group. An editorial addressing the issue of complications pointed out that these findings should not prevent the use of testosterone in appropriate cases, but caution should be exercised.[16] It is up to the physician to determine what is appropriate.

Identifying older men who are androgen deficient includes those who complain of poor morning erections, low sexual drive, erectile dysfunction, physical weakness, fatigue, and depression. One study concluded that only three complaints, the sexual symptoms mentioned above, correlated with a low serum testosterone level.[17] Other symptoms, such as limited physical strength, loss of energy, or fatigue, may or may not be related to low testosterone. The authors of this study concluded there is "substantial overlap between late-onset hypogonadism and non-specific symptoms of aging."[18]

In an attempt to define the level of testosterone needed to account for lean body mass, muscle strength, and sexual function, 198 men underwent pharmacological treatment with drugs that eliminated testosterone and the conversion of testosterone to estradiol.[19] Then, by administering testosterone, the specific dose of testosterone required to maintain a particular function could be determined. Testosterone deficiency accounted for a decrease in lean body mass, thigh muscle area, leg strength, and sexual desire. Lean body mass, thigh muscle area, and erectile function were reduced at a testosterone dose that provided only 200 nanograms/dl. This level was clearly in the hypogonadal range, and the dose of testosterone needed to correct these deficiencies would have to be increased to provide a more effective dose. The authors concluded that "testosterone supplements seem justified in men with testosterone in this range."[20] Even testosterone values in the 250–300 ng/dl range are borderline, and a therapeutic goal would be to provide a dose that would raise the testosterone to a level at which the symptoms remitted.[21]

What should an elderly man do who is diagnosed as having a low testosterone? Assume his complaints are loss of energy, decreased physical strength, and a loss of libido. Should he risk taking testosterone, either by injection or by a gel, which is absorbed through the skin when rubbed over the upper arm and shoulders? There have been "highly publicized reports" about the cardiac risks in testosterone use.[22] These reports are outweighed by data from other studies indicating no change or even improvement in cardiac risk.[23] Some evidence indicates that men with low testosterone have a greater risk for heart attack and stroke. These seemingly conflicting data leave a patient in a quandary as to whether or not to start on testosterone. One possible explanation for the increased risk of heart attack could be that in men taking testosterone and regaining physical strength, the increased physical activity may precipitate a heart attack. Screening for heart disease prior to starting testosterone seems prudent, along with treating hypertension and high cholesterol.

One side effect of testosterone treatment is to increase the hematocrit (percentage of red blood cells in the circulation).[24] If the hematocrit rises to a dangerous level, the testosterone dose may have to be reduced or eliminated. An elevated hematocrit approaching 60 percent may lead to vascular congestion and predispose to a stroke. In a recent study of 300 men receiving testosterone, about a third had an elevated red blood cell count after two years.[25] In this same report, there were five cases of prostate cancer diagnosed. This is actually higher than would be expected in the general population. Still, older men being considered for testosterone therapy should have their prostate examined and a baseline PSA done. A relatively rapid rise in the PSA after a year should alert the treating physician to the possibility of prostate cancer.

The Gland Illusion

As previously noted, one of the effects of testosterone on the body is the muscle-building function. As Charles Atlas noted years ago, the desire to add muscle to a man's torso is almost universal. In addition to testosterone itself, there are several other synthetic derivatives termed anabolic steroids which accentuate the muscle-building attribute of testosterone and have been used to treat patients suffering from burns, certain cancer therapies, and muscle-wasting diseases.[26] The alteration in the chemical structure of the synthetic androgens affects the metabolism of the drug, and caution should be used in long-term use because of possible liver damage.

The use of testosterone and its derivatives in athletics gained popularity in the Olympic Games during the Cold War, and has continued to the present time.[27] A crude attempt to use the secretion from the testicle in sports was mentioned in the first chapter, when James Galvin, a baseball pitcher, was given an injection of a testicular emulsion in hopes of improving his performance. Recently, a supplier of anabolic steroids was charged in federal court with distributing steroids to "high-school and professional athletes."[28] This indicates the lure of enhanced performance from drugs, particularly anabolic steroids, remains in our society.

The adverse consequences of excess androgenic stimulation include decreased production of sperm, acne, hypertension, changes in blood lipids associated with atherosclerosis, and previously mentioned increased red blood cell production above the upper limit of normal. In women, the masculinizing effect produces deepening of the voice, clitoral hypertrophy, menstrual irregularities, and increased facial hair.[29] Women also are subject to some of the same adverse effects as men.[30]

In recent years, popular news magazines have featured articles on aging and low testosterone.[31] The symptoms of decreased muscle mass and strength, decreased libido, erectile dysfunction, fatigue, and increased abdominal fat are described, and the fact that testosterone levels fall with age are presented. Anecdotal evidence is presented describing the improvement in the above symptoms after testosterone treatment. However, there are warnings mentioned about possible adverse consequences. In addition to the previously mentioned adverse effects, sleep apnea was mentioned as developing or worsening with testosterone treatment.

11. *Testosterone*

With an aging population and the expected increase in testosterone replacement therapy, the question of who should receive the hormone will require judicious appraisal on the part of patient and physician. There is a place for testosterone treatment. The need should be based on the patient's complaints and a demonstrated low serum testosterone. In a recent article published by the American Urological Association (AUA), the benefits and risks of testosterone treatment are presented.[32] The issue of cardiovascular safety was raised and two recent articles reporting increased cardiovascular risk were discussed. In the opinion of one author, the studies on cardiovascular risk contained flaws in methodology, which made statistical analysis inconclusive.[33] The other study on cardiovascular risks was withdrawn because of numerous complaints. The summation of the AUA article was that erectile problems may not respond to testosterone therapy but improved strength, energy, cognition, mood, and quality of life have been credited with testosterone therapy in appropriate hypogonadal cases.

Another author counseled against testosterone use, pointing out the symptoms of decreased energy, decreased motivation, and sleep disturbance may or may not be caused by testosterone deficiency. Based on complaints alone, 25 percent of men diagnosed with supposed hypogonadism never had a serum testosterone measured, suggesting some degree of overuse of testosterone to treat certain general complaints. The author concludes, "Until a large prospective, multicenter, long-term, longitudinal study is conducted on testosterone replacement therapy, there should be a prudent tincture of caution and acknowledgement that there are known and unknown concerns with testosterone treatment."[34] There should be no problem in prescribing testosterone in men with complaints suggesting low testosterone *plus* a documented low testosterone, and if treatment is started, careful monitoring should be done.

Recently, the pros and cons of testosterone replacement therapy were presented in the *New England Journal of Medicine*.[35] As an example of a man who might be considered a candidate for testosterone, a sixty-one-year-old presented to his physician complaining of erectile dysfunction and a lack of energy, which affected his tennis game. This man was interested in knowing what his testosterone level was. Possibly the man had been watching television commercials depicting an individual with similar complaints. His physician ordered the test and the result was 275 ng/dl. This value was slightly below the lower limit of normal. His symptoms were not atypical of men with hypogonadism, but the loss of libido and erectile function were most important to him. Before starting testosterone, a digital rectal examination and PSA level were done, which were normal. If a decision was to be made to start testosterone, the patient should be appraised of the possible risks. Although prostate cancer may occur in a man taking testosterone, the medical literature does not indicate the risk is high. This individual was started on testosterone and an evaluation was done after six months to see if the symptoms which brought him to the doctor were resolved. If so, then therapy may be continued, with monitoring for any adverse effects.

A contrary view was presented, which questioned whether his symptoms were related to androgen deficiency or related to aging.[36] One recommendation was to encourage the patient to lose weight, since he could afford to shed some pounds. This would likely improve his tennis game. His decreased libido and erectile dysfunction might or might not respond to testosterone therapy because, although his testosterone level was below the lower limit of normal, he did not have a level low enough for erectile dysfunction to be an expected consequence. But as the article pointed out, "High quality data regarding both benefit and risk of testosterone-replacement treatment in this age group are limited." There are still unanswered questions regarding cardiovascular safety in men taking testosterone.

In 2015, a summary of a recent FDA meeting on the risks of testosterone replacement was published.[37] The meeting was prompted by relatively recent publications on the cardiovascular risks of testosterone replacement. An advisory panel concluded that the use of testosterone should be limited to those with primary hypogonadism and not those with age-related decline in testosterone. Also, labeling of testosterone products should include a warning about cardiovascular risk. The safety of testosterone therapy requires more study to document its safety and who might be at risk.

Recently, however, the initial results of a study of the effects of testosterone treatment in older men sponsored by the National Institute of Health was reported in the *New England Journal of Medicine*.[38] The participants in the study were at least sixty-five, the average age was seventy-two, and the testosterone level was 275 ng/deciliter or lower. Almost 90 percent of the participants were white, most were overweight, and about a third had diabetes. The study lasted one year.

The results showed that in these older men there was some improvement in sexual function, although the improvement lessened in the last three months of the study (significance?). There was also slight improvement in mood and a lower severity of depressive symptoms. Slight improvement was noted in physical performance.

In regard to adverse events, 23 out of 394 participants were found to have a rise of 1 ng/ml or greater over the course of the study. One man who had received testosterone was diagnosed with prostate cancer, and one man in the placebo group also developed prostate cancer. In a follow-up period the next year, three more men were diagnosed with prostate cancer in the testosterone group and one in the placebo group. Cardiovascular events, myocardial infarction or stroke, occurred in seven men in the testosterone group and seven in the placebo group.

Because the report of the study covered one year, it is difficult to draw any long-term conclusions.[39] Does the sexual improvement persist during treatment for a longer period of time? Is there a slightly greater risk of developing prostate cancer with continued testosterone use? Are there an increased number of cardiovascular events with continued testosterone treatment? These are some of the issues a longer study with more subjects should further define.

12

The Fountain of Youth

O for one hour of youthful joy!
Give me back my twentieth spring!
I'd rather laugh a bright-haired boy
Than reign a gray-haired king!
—Oliver Wendell Holmes

"Water is good: it benefits all things and does not compete with them."
—Lao Tzu 600 BCE

If the reader is somewhat diffident about whether he or she should take hormones to recapture youth or stave off the consequences of old age, consider the fountain of youth, or fountains of youth, since there are multiple sites claiming to have waters that have a history of easing the ailments associated with aging.[1]

"Nobody knows exactly when the idea of immortality-inducing waters first trickled into consciousness," concluded Adam Gollner.[2] For centuries, there had been accounts of healing waters, whether from a fountain, mineral spring, lake, or river. Drinking the water or bathing in it would restore the benefits of youth. The healing waters of mineral baths have been considered a source of rejuvenation, dating back to Roman times; the term spa is an acronym for the Roman words "salus per aquam," meaning health by water.[3] Stories of a fountain of youth emerged from India, carried by explorers who claimed to have witnessed such sources or heard tales from locals who claimed to be one hundred years old.[4] In Europe, Lucas Cranach painted a fountain of youth (see frontispiece) at the age of seventy-four, prior to his demise in 1553. In a sense, it represents his last testament to his view of life.[5] The painting shows a statue of Venus and Cupid in the middle of a pool surrounding the fountain. They are meant to convey the idea that the pool represents a "font of love." Frail, elderly women are shown arriving by stretcher and wheelbarrow, and being carried to the pool. They enter the water on the left where they are attended to, and as the rejuvenating waters transform them, they emerge on the right, appearing youthful again. After leaving the pool, the young ladies are escorted to a tent where they don fashionable clothing and proceed to a table where food and beverage await them. From there they join a dance in progress. In the lower right corner of the painting, a man and woman are partly hidden by vegetation and appear to be engaged in conversation, perhaps leading to an amorous adventure.

As exploration of the New World continued, several sources of magical waters were reported. The east coast of Florida was one site, the Bahamas another, at or near an island now owned by the magician/ illusionist David Copperfield.[6] The Spanish explorer Ponce de Leon is generally credited with discovering and attempting to settle the east coast of Florida, first in 1513 and then in 1521.[7] The attempt at establishing a settlement in what he named Florida was thwarted by natives from the Timucua tribe, who drove Ponce de Leon and his men from the Florida coast to Cuba. It was there that Ponce de Leon died from a wound suffered in the fight with the natives.

Although Ponce de Leon was believed to have been looking for a fountain of youth, there was no mention of this in the authorization of the expedition by King Ferdinand of Spain. He was to look for land to colonize, gold, and a possible source for slaves. It wasn't until 1535 that Gonzalo de Oviedo, writing the history of the West Indies, claimed that Ponce de Leon was seeking a fountain of youth on the waters off Bimini to cure his impotence.[8] This may have been an assumption by Oviedo, based on gossip circulating in the Spanish Court.

In 1565, Pedro Mendez de Aviles established a colony at or near the current site of St. Augustine, Florida.[9] That site, along with several others, has claimed to have a fountain of youth. But it wasn't until the nineteenth century that tourists began to visit Florida, when the railroad was built along Florida's east coast. Recently, a reporter for the *New York Times* visited several of the sites claiming to have a fountain of youth. Punta Gorda, Florida, has claimed to have such a site for more than one hundred years. The reporter located what passed for a "Fountain of Youth," a "blocky little drinking fountain ... covered with green tile that must have been decorative ninety years ago but was now cracked and stained."[10] Opening the spigot brought forth water that smelled "sulfurous." An accompanying sign warned that the water "exceeds the maximum contamination for radioactivity as determined by the United States Environmental Protection Agency." It is fortunate that some quack hasn't bottled the water and sold it as a rejuvenating radioactive tonic.

Further down the road, about a half hour's drive, was another site, called Warm Mineral Springs. Here a sign indicated this was "Ponce de Leon's Original Fountain of Youth."[11] The site consisted of a large pool of water nourished by a warm salty spring. Some sixty years ago, the spring and pool had been a popular health spa complete with restaurant and a massage salon. Today the facilities are closed, although the pool is still open for swimming.

Two other sites along Florida's west coast have claimed to have a fountain of youth.[12] One was located near Ocala, Florida. In the later nineteenth century, Ocala became a tourist destination. Steamboat rides on the nearby waterways provided tourists with views of wildlife and lush tropical vegetation. With the advent of glass-bottom boats, visitors could also observe colorful fish and reptiles. This area also became famous for a time as a site for filming Tarzan movies. More recently, parts of the James Bond films *Thunderball* and *Moonraker* were shot there. Ocala and the surrounding region are now well known for raising thoroughbred racehorses. Alas, the site of the magical fountain has been lost.

The other site for a fountain of youth on the west Florida coast is in St. Petersburg. Here a slightly more developed site bore the title "Fountain of Youth."[13] The fountain is white, pentagonally shaped, and with a large stainless-steel tap that delivers a stream of clear, odorless water. The reporter for the *Times* sensed that the water may have come from the "city's regular water supply." But perhaps it still has some youth-inducing properties. It would take a demographer to determine if the inhabitants of St. Petersburg really do live longer. Up to this point, the sites mentioned are all on the west coast of Florida.

The current site which claims to have the original fountain of youth is St. Augustine, Florida.[14] It was Henry Flagler, former partner of John D. Rockefeller, whose Florida and East Coast Railroad helped put St. Augustine on the map. He wanted to make St. Augustine a winter resort similar to what Newport, Rhode Island, was in the summer. Flagler constructed two large hotels and acquired a third, so that by the 1890s, St. Augustine had become a thriving community. An alligator farm opened in 1893 and this became an additional tourist attraction. A directory of St. Augustine in 1885 made no mention of a fountain of youth. A 1904 series of pictures of St. Augustine shows no scene of a fountain of youth, suggesting the fountain had not yet become a major attraction in the town.[15]

It wasn't until the arrival of Diamond Lil in 1900, who purchased property in St. Augustine on which there was a spring, that a Fountain of Youth was promoted.[16] Lil arrived from the Klondike gold mining region, with a diamond in a front tooth, expensive-appearing jewelry, and an entrepreneurial spirit. She began selling "Fountain of Youth" water for twenty-five cents a glass. The discovery of an old cross and a few human bones near the fountain reinforced her belief that this was the original site of Ponce de Leon's landing. The fountain remained her property until she died in an automobile accident. The property was then acquired by the Walter B. Fraser family, who maintain the Fountain of Youth and hold a copyright on Ponce de Leon Fountain of Youth Water.[17]

A trip to St. Augustine has its rejuvenating aspects: the warm, balmy sea breezes, the semi-tropical foliage, and the excited visitors enjoying the surroundings. There are fifteen acres devoted to the memory of the Spanish settlement on the Florida east coast. This archeological park, as it is termed, includes the fountain, a reproduction of a Spanish watchtower, a reconstructed First Mission Church, which was first built in 1587, a historically correct example of a Timucuan Indian village, a pavilion where special events such as weddings are held, and, of course, a gift shop, where Fountain of Youth Water is for sale. The park is well-maintained and free from graffiti and fast-food litter. The actual fountain has a spigot attached and is an enclosed area. Visitors line up to partake of the water—plastic cups are provided. Some of the visitors, particularly women, were photographing each other as part of a before and after exercise, hoping at some point to see if there was any improvement in their appearance. On sampling the water, I found it odorless and tasteless. It could have come from the city water source. There were no canes or crutches lying around the fountain, which might imply a rapid recovery from some debilitating condition. A less honorable establishment might have left an empty wheelchair near the fountain, indicating a miraculous recovery had resulted from imbibing the water from the fountain. The gift shop in the park sold a variety of items, hats, T-shirts, mugs, and bottles of water from the Ponce de Leon Fountain of Youth for those wishing an additional rejuvenating boost after returning home.

But are the Fountain of Youth and the archeological park the actual site where Ponce de Leon landed and identified the fountain? There are numerous skeptics, as Adam Gollner discovered.[18] Some years ago, the St. Augustine Historical Society issued this opinion: "There is no fountain of youth, as we all know, and it is silly and quacky to carry on the invention of a woman [Diamond Lil] who was not in her right mind."[19] A visit to the St. Augustine Historical Archives provides "filing cabinets" containing various arguments as to the possible location of the youth-inducing fountain. Those interested can make up their own mind as to the authenticity of the Fountain.

Perhaps it is just as well that the Fountain of Youth remains something of a mystery, just as the countless means of regaining lost youth have a mysterious quality, an indefiniteness, unless, as Mark Twain wrote, "the faith is strong."

13

Direct-to-Consumer Advertising

> "You can tell the ideals of a nation by its advertising."
> —Norman Douglas, *South Wind* (1917)

John R. Brinkley was a master at directing his advertising to a receptive public. In the early years of his goat gland practice in Milford, Kansas, he relied on pamphlets sent through the mail to prospective patients, informing them about his rejuvenating surgery. This printed material also informed the recipient about traveling to Milford by road or train. In another form letter, he would boast, "I believe that I am here for the purpose of performing surgery, advanced surgery, and curative surgery. I believe that my surgical work is fifty years ahead of its time when it comes to curing insanity, diseases of old age and assisting bright minds and valuable men and women to remain here and finish work of value [for] the coming generation."[1] Addressing a frequent problem among his listening audience, he wrote, "If you are sexually weak or interested in matters concerning sex for yourself or your wife, we have some sound advice concerning this."[2] A visit to Milford would provide that advice. Brinkley was not shy about approaching members of the press. In an undated letter to the managing editor of the *Chicago Tribune*, he wrote, "My work appeals chiefly to brain-workers, and it is not surprising therefore that so many prominent people in the newspaper business should have availed themselves of my service."[3] Brinkley may have been referring to his visit to Los Angeles, at which time he performed goat testicle surgery on two of the editors of the *Los Angeles Times*.

If an individual inquired by mail about Brinkley's practice but had

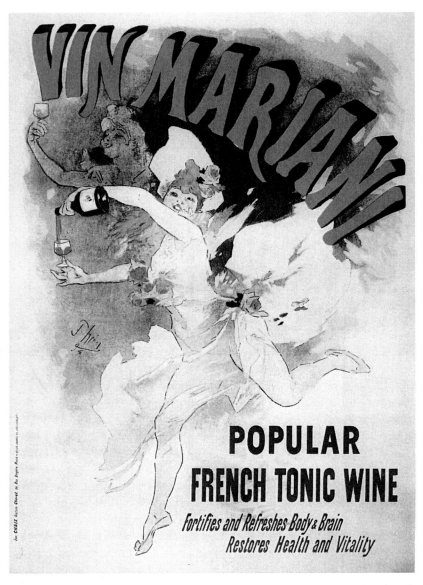

This enticing poster produced by Jules Chéret, in 1894, represents an excellent example of letting the picture capture the consumer's attention. Angelo Mariani successfully marketed this wine up to the start of the First World War. The fact that the wine contained cocaine probably added to its popularity. The English text indicated the product was for the North American and British market. (Courtesy of Dr. William H. Helfand, *Health for Sale*, Philadelphia Museum of Art/Yale University Press, 2011.)

not followed through by making an appointment to visit Milford, he could expect the following letter: "Just what kind of a fellow are you? You wrote to us for information regarding our work and we sent it to you. Evidently you are not satisfied with your present state of health or you would not be making such inquiries.... Now, after we have sent you literature and have written you, we can't even hear from you. To us this means that you ARE interested and it is up to us to write the kind of letter that you will answer. That's what we are trying to do now."[4] The recipient of such a letter could expect several more cajoling letters from Brinkley.

But it was Brinkley's use of the radio that provided him with a highly successful avenue to reach prospective patients. He achieved such financial success that he could acquire expensive automobiles and an airplane, and eventually run for governor of Kansas. Brinkley founded KFKB in 1922, and with his use of radio, he was able to reach thousands, then hundreds of thousands of listeners, as more of the population acquired radios. As a reporter for the *Kansas City Star* wrote, "Brinkley's ballyhoo is in his radio lectures each day. In these, he describes the ailments of men, the symptoms of lost manhood, and the sure remedy he has in his goat gland operation. He invites correspondence through the mails. Once a person writes to Brinkley, he is doomed from then on to receive a deluge of pamphlets, testimonials and urgings to go to Milford to be examined."[5] A goat gland implant usually followed.

Once Brinkley had established his radio station, almost every letter he sent out made reference to his lectures on health issues. In these lectures, Brinkley could be quite persuasive and was regarded as one of the first "radio personalities." His station KFKB was declared the most popular radio station in America, based on a poll done by a radio magazine in 1930.[6] When the U.S. State Department began to monitor his broadcasts from Mexico, where he started a radio station after losing his radio license in the U.S., a State Department listener concluded that Brinkley had "an arresting and highly magnetic radio personality which radiates confidence, faith, and sincerity."[7] A local doctor in Kansas, no fan of Brinkley, conceded that "his voice was pleasant and his style of delivery was directed in a very personal manner at the listener."[8]

Brinkley could be regarded as the man who, perhaps more than any other, foresaw the great potential of radio as an advertising medium. In the early days of radio, advertising as a means of supporting the station was controversial; yet Brinkley carried out an advertising campaign directly to the public that set a standard at the time.[9]

But Brinkley was hardly the first practitioner to make his services known to the public. Drug makers, medicine men, bone setters, midwives, faith healers, herbalists, and witch doctors had been making their presence known for centuries by word of mouth or stone tablets. The invention of the printing press resulted in spreading the knowledge of medical practitioners and apothecaries to the public. In sixteenth-century England, in an attempt to control the practice of medicine, the Royal College of Physicians was created.[10] King Henry VIII banned medical practice by the clergy about this time. In 1618, the *London Pharmacopoeia* was published in Latin, the language of the educated physician.[11] But with its subsequent translation into English, an untold number of unorthodox practitioners were able to formulate remedies from herbs, animal parts, and minerals. Apothecaries knew what the members of the College were prescribing for their patients and would concoct a similar product to sell directly to the public. Gradually, advertisements by apothecaries began to appear in newspapers and handbills. A public demand for medical advice and products emerged. From 1688 to 1711, there were an estimated two hundred printers and sellers of medical works.[12]

By 1700, about half of England's population was literate, and with the spread of medical knowledge, every man and woman could be his or her own doctor.[13] A person wishing to rejuvenate himself or herself had no shortage of sources of medical information. During this period, more women became medical practitioners. After all, they were the ones who cared for the sick at home. They often maintained an herb garden and would exchange ideas with other women as to what worked to calm a fever. Some recipe books also contained information for the preparation of various home remedies.[14]

The advent of coffeehouses provided a site for the free exchange of medical advice among the patrons.[15] The walls of these establishments were said to be papered with advertisements for practitioners, apothecaries, and surgeons. Unfortunately, this practice allowed quacks and various imposters to advertise their services as well.

In 1624, the term "patent medicine" came about by the passage of the Statute of Monopolies.[16] This allowed the exclusive production of a new product over a fourteen-year period. The contents of the product need not be disclosed so as to prevent fraudulent duplication. However, these patents were often ignored by various practitioners, apothecaries, and quacks, who guessed what was in the product and attempted to reproduce and market it under a new name. Today the term patent medicine applies to a nonprescription product protected by a trademark.

Exploration of the world resulted in the introduction of new products into the medical marketplace. Nutmeg, cloves, and cinnamon became part of medical products.[17] One justification for the new medical products was the quote from the Apocrypha, Ecclesiasticus (Sirach) 38:4: "The Lord hath created medicines of the earth and he that is wise will not abhor them." By the eighteenth century, the College of Physicians was threatened by the growing competition of quacks, chemists, apothecaries, and even surgeons who were gaining a living by marketing various "cure-alls," containing some of the new ingredients.[18] The many botanical cures that became available to the public in the early nineteenth century led to the phrase "every man his physician."[19] In an attempt to define who was and who wasn't a physician in the United States, the American Medical Association was founded in 1847. Consequently, a person calling himself a physician and a member of the AMA would be recognized as having received more training and acquired more expertise in treating various ailments.

Recall that when Brown-Séquard reported his self-injection of the testicular emulsion, word spread quickly to other countries. Success varied, but it seemed there was no shortage of volunteers eager to duplicate the rejuvenating qualities of the product. Manufacturers of patent medicines used the gland idea to produce a variety of products aimed at rejuvenating the aging male. In 1906, a forerunner of the Food and Drug Administration was created during the Teddy Roosevelt administration.[20] This agency required that a drug had to list the ingredients and strength, and to assure purity. Misbranding or misleading labels were subject to a fine or jail time. But "patent medicines" went unchecked for the most part. It was difficult to tell what was a legitimate drug and what wasn't. In 1938, the Pure Food and Drug Act was amended so that a drug had to be deemed safe, and required instructions on how to administer the product. Amid the many health care products on the market, the AMA Council on Pharmacy and Chemistry made the distinction between patent medicines and drugs that required a doctor's prescription. Up to this point, medical advertising was overseen by the Federal Trade Commission (FTC). Then in 1962, the Kefauver-Harris Amendment required the manufacturer to prove the safety and efficacy of a medical product. Drug trials would require the patient's informed consent. And the FDA, not the FTC, would regulate the advertising of prescription drugs.[21] Advertising would be aimed at physicians, not the general public.

In 1997, pressured by the advertising and pharmaceutical industries, the FDA permitted advertising of prescription drugs.[22] This action allowed the complete armamentarium of advertising methods to be directed at the consumer/patient. Among these methods was direct mail, which focused on persuading the recipient to request a new product or send in a reply card, which would ensure receiving additional information.[23] A print ad in a newspaper or magazine is another method aimed at capturing the attention of the reader. The key elements of the ad are the illustration(s), the headline or bold statement within the ad designed to capture the interest of the reader, the message itself, and instructions on where to call or write for more information.[24]

As Dr. Brinkley found, radio has the potential to reach a wide audience, although in recent years, certain stations will aim a message at a particular audience such as teenagers, a more sophisticated audience interested in financial news, or classical music enthusiasts. By 1938, radio had surpassed print in generating advertising revenue.[25] To be effective, radio ads require active listening. "The first five seconds are important."[26] To sustain interest, there is usually background music or certain sound effects relative to the product being advertised. For a sixty-second commercial, the message should tell what the product is, what the strong points are, and how the product (drug) is better than other similar products. Then the ad signs off with a reminder name or theme. A song or slogan should stick in the listener's ear. A shorter ad still needs these components to be effective.

In the last sixty years, television has become the most important source of information directed at the consumer.[27] It generally has a broad appeal, but may target audiences within a certain geographic area served by a local medical center. Television may also target certain audiences such as housewives or senior citizens experiencing problems associated with aging. In television, the visual as well as the audio work to drive home the message that the product being shown will make the audience healthier, younger looking, and more physically attractive.

A good TV commercial for a pharmaceutical product will combine promotion, information, and entertainment.[28] The narrator may or may not be identified. If the spokesperson is a celebrity, he or she will provide the dialogue. There may be fear instilled in the viewer by phrases such as "you may have" or "don't wait any longer." The message and background music are generally upbeat so that, despite fear or concern, the consumer will proceed to schedule an appointment with a doctor. The ads may contain certain less definitive phrases such as "gets more out of" or "with fewer symptoms." These are some of the parts of a successful TV ad that will motivate you to see your doctor about a particular product.

The FDA allows three different types of prescription drug advertisements: (1) Product Claim. Here the name of the drug is provided along with benefits and risks. The claim must not be misleading and must be easily understandable; (2) Reminder Advertisement. The ad simply mentions the name of the drug. It assumes the listener or reader already knows about the drug's use. An antacid would be an example. The ad cannot suggest anything further about use or risks; (3) Help-Seeking Advertisement. The ad describes a disease or condition but does not recommend or suggest a specific drug treatment. An example would be an elevated cholesterol.[29]

For print ads, the drug's benefits and most serious risks are presented in the main body of the ad, in keeping with risk disclosure requirements. The less important risks are presented in smaller print as a brief summary. Product Claim and Reminder print ads must include the statement, "You are encouraged to report negative side effects to the FDA." Phone 1–800-FDA-1088.[30]

Radio and TV may make statements about the drug's benefits and the most important risk information. The time taken by the ad limits more detailed information about side effects and risks. The ad may include every risk, at times spoken rapidly, or provide information about where the listener can obtain further knowledge about the drug.

The FDA provides some questions that a consumer/patient should consider before inquiring about a particular medication.[31] First, what is the disease or condition that the drug in question treats and why do I think I may have the condition? Assuming that the patient has this condition, is he part of the population the drug is approved to treat? For example, if a person has mild Type II diabetes and is managing it with diet and exercise, starting a drug that he has seen advertised could expose him to undesirable side effects and not improve control of his diabetes.

How will this drug affect other medications I am taking? Will certain foods, beverages, or vitamins affect the action of the drug? Some drugs will interfere with each other and possibly lead to undesirable side effects.

Are there other medications for this condition, and are there generic, less costly forms of this drug? Do other drugs for this condition have the same risks?

What else can I do to help or treat the condition? For osteoporosis, exercise, increasing calcium intake, and vitamin D may be an appropriate approach.

Finally, how can a patient learn more about his condition and a drug that he believes may help him? Consulting his physician is one way. Another is to enter the name of the condition or drug on a Web site. Drug companies provide information about their products, although some may regard this information as biased in favor of their product. Books are available, such as home health guides or the *Physician's Desk Reference* (*PDR*), which will offer information about a particular drug. Various support groups have information on the disease in question, assuming it is a recognized disease or condition, and not simply symptoms that the patient believes may represent a serious disease. Vising a support group may provide the opportunity to ask members about the drug in question, but expect to get variable responses, some favorable and others less so. Some may even say the drug made them worse!

Drug companies believe that direct advertising to the public is to the consumer/patient's benefit. Their advertising is approved by the FDA and they believe their information is accurate. The advertisement may have alerted a consumer about certain symptoms that were ignored but could represent a serious illness.

The cost of direct-to-consumer advertising of prescription products is not insignificant. Spending on pharmaceutical marketing grew from $11.4 billion in 1997 to $29.9 billion in 2005.[32] During this period, violations in the advertising determined by the FDA fell from 142 in 1997 to 21 in 2005. This can be interpreted as indicating pharmaceutical companies and their ad agencies produced more accurate and informative ads, or that the FDA was lax in enforcing regulations. Not surprisingly, the majority of the complaints about misleading ads were submitted by rival drug companies.

In 2004, a survey was done by the FDA about physicians' acceptance of direct-to-consumer advertising (DTCA). This was seven years after DTCA had been approved by the FDA. Fifty-three percent of the respondents thought that direct advertising to the public contributed to better questions being asked about a particular product and facilitated an easier conversation about various drugs. In some cases it encouraged the adherence to the patient's current medications rather than embark on a new, possibly dangerous treatment. It also reduced the underdiagnosis and treatment of certain conditions, when a patient could define more clearly to his doctor how he felt after seeing a certain ad. Advertising also reduced the stigma associated with certain illnesses, such as depression or cancer, since an individual could see or read about a patient with a similar condition. Most physicians tended to agree that ads led patients to believe the drug in question was more effective than the ad indicated. In some instances, physicians felt pressure to prescribe a particular brand name drug when the patient mentioned the drug. However, only eight percent of physicians felt "very pressured" when a patient requested a particular medication. Finally, eighty-two percent of physicians believed their patients understood that only their doctor can decide whether or not a particular drug is right for them.[33]

Through DTCA, the public has been made aware of various conditions about which they may or may not have been aware and may not have impacted their lives. These include restless legs, erectile dysfunction, sleep disorders, social anxiety disorder, stomach acid reflux, metabolic syndrome, low testosterone ("low T"), atrial fibrillation ("A fib"), urinary frequency, and new immunotherapy for certain types of cancer.[34] Knowledge of these conditions may prompt a visit to a doctor's office to discuss the problem and possibly obtain a prescription for a new, expensive medication.

In 2000, the top fifteen drugs in advertising revenue accounted for fifty-four percent of direct-to-consumer advertisements. These were for chronic conditions including allergy, asthma, elevated cholesterol, arthritis, depression, obesity, and erectile dysfunction.[35] None of these are life-threatening, but all reflect the need to control or eliminate a condition and regain good health, in a sense, a rejuvenation.

Dr. Marcia Angell, former editor of the *New England Journal of Medicine*, has criticized pharmaceutical companies for the amount of money spent on advertising vs. the amount spent on research and development of new drugs.[36] The ads are more about selling a drug than informing the consumer. In a subsequent publication, she warns about the relationship between drug companies, academia, and health care professionals.[37] Doctors have had favors bestowed upon them for supporting a certain drug. A doctor's endorsement and use of the drug may have been influenced by a trip to a vacation site paid for by a drug company in return for a lecture to a group of physicians in support of a certain drug. Dr. Angell notes that medical literature involving drugs rarely compares one drug with another, but compares it to a placebo. Another criticism of the drug industry is that there are too many "me too" drugs, products that are very similar to another on the market and hold only a slight, if any, advantage over other medications for the same condition, some being available in generic form.

There have been several books written about the pharmaceutical industry this past decade and its influence on the consumer/patient. In one book, the authors question how much a patient really understands how the medication works.[38] In any given week, eighty-one percent of adults in the U.S. take at least one medication, and nearly a third of these will take as many as five different drugs.[39] It is hoped that the patients have some understanding what the drugs are treating. The cost of advertising these drugs is projected to be $11.4 billion by 2017. This advertising will more than likely result in more new expensive drugs being prescribed, thus adding to the cost of medical care.

It isn't just known illnesses that are being targeted but the "medicalization" of certain symptoms that are magnified in the patient's mind.[40] What actions are taken when a patient believes he has a problem, based on an advertisement? One study showed that thirty-nine percent of patients exposed to advertising made an appointment with their doctor. Thirty-six percent obtained an over-the-counter product for their symptoms. The remainder either resumed or refilled a medication they had previously taken for the condition or persisted in questioning their doctor about a new drug and, in some cases, obtained a new prescription.[41]

Another analysis of the consumer response to direct-to-consumer advertising revealed that fifty-one percent of respondents had no interest in health messages conveyed by advertising.[42] Twenty-eight percent discussed the newly discovered drug with their physician but deferred to the advice of their physician about starting on the drug. There were thirteen percent who decided to obtain an over-the-counter drug for their condition. Lastly, there were eight percent who persisted in their quest for the new medication and presumably obtained it. They are the "solution seekers," who are usually overmedicated.

Some authors on the subject of medical advertising acknowledge there are patients with well-documented illnesses, but in their opinion, many advertisements are meant to convey to the patient that he has a condition which might be improved by a different or newly advertised drug. And "too much ordinary life" is turned into a medical condition.[43] Disappointment becomes depression.

Some authors maintain that too many guidelines written by experts in the field are influenced by big pharmaceutical firms.[44] Rather than accept current guidelines on the danger of elevated cholesterol, the authors are skeptical on the recommendations to lower it with medication. This will come as a surprise to physicians, particularly cardiologists, who accept the research showing the danger of high cholesterol in contributing to cardiovascular disease, heart attack and stroke.[45] These same authors cite an "authority" who accepts a systolic blood pressure of 160 mm Hg, clearly in the hypertensive range. This ignores American Heart Association guidelines which indicate that normal blood pressure is 120/80. Pre-hypertensive range is 120–139/80–90mm Hg. Hypertension stage 1 is 140–159/90–99 and stage 2 is 160/100. Sustained high blood pressure is an invitation to a heart attack or stroke.[46] Anyone ignoring these generally accepted guidelines is at risk.

Attention deficit disorder (ADD) is another condition which lends itself to potential overtreatment.[47] Here, disordered learning, inattention, disruptive behavior, and hyperactivity are the characteristics. But for some children, boredom with the material being taught and the need to get up and move about may represent behavior which some believe should be treated with medication. A health care professional may find a home situation or cultural factors contributing to the perceived problem. And the child/young adult may be of superior intelligence and find the classroom material quite dull. Use of amphetamine-like drugs has been recommended by advertisements as a solution to getting a child to improve his school behavior and performance.[48] Possibly, improving a child's study habits or correcting rowdy behavior are just as effective as a drug.

In an effort to promote the use of the antidepressant Paxil, a special ailment called social anxiety disorder was created.[49] Certainly everyone has experienced some level of anxiety before a presentation to a group or joining a party where you are not familiar with any of the guests. But these situations are usually overcome by most of us without resorting to drugs. Granted, there are individuals who seem to suffer extraordinary anxiety to the point where their voices tremble or their hands shake. In such situations, seeking the help of a mental health professional may be preferable to taking a drug, with the risk of side effects or becoming dependent on the drug.

Another condition for which medication is sometimes advertised is irritable bowel syndrome (IBS), characterized by irregular bowel habits, diarrhea and/or constipation.[50] There are patients with frequent bowel movements who are found to have Crohn's Disease, an inflammation of the bowel. This condition is treated with specific medication designed to quiet bowel activity. But for those who simply have irregular bowel habits, dietary measures, regulating fluid intake, reducing caffeine intake, and over-the-counter medication may suffice.

Premenstrual tension or premenstrual syndrome is experienced by many women. An extreme form of this syndrome has been labeled "premenstrual dysphoric disorder."[51] This disorder has been characterized by cyclical mood shifts, anxiety, and, in some cases, abdominal pain. According to the above source, this disorder occurs in only about seven percent of women, but an antidepressant has been marketed as a means of coping with this problem. The problem lies in who actually experiences this "disorder," and is it appropriate to start on an antidepressant, which may have to be taken for an indefinite period, with the potential risks of long-term medication?

Carl Elliot has written about what he terms "enhancement technology" provided by pharmaceutical agents.[52] An example is anti-anxiety drugs targeting individuals who want to feel reassured and more confident. Another word used to convince the consumer that he needs a particular medication is "self-fulfilment."[53] Here the consumer needs to be convinced that he hasn't lived up to his expectations and somehow needs to make use of his talents, which heretofore have not been manifested in his life. An example is an advertisement that shows a man giving a business report. There appears to be a warm, friendly atmosphere surrounding the presentation, but inwardly, the presenter is suffering profound anxiety.[54] Will the anxiety be detected by members of the audience? This anxiety might detract from the message being presented. A drug might relieve the feeling of anxiety and improve the quality of the presentation. True social phobia is a more extreme form of shyness. The message of the above scenario is to take medication that will curtail this condition. One pharmaceutical firm uses the phrase, "Relieve the anxiety and reveal the real person." The "extrovert is frozen within you."[55]

Another example in which DTCA was used to promote an anti-anxiety drug is the phrase, "I got my playfulness back with drug—."[56] Here the appeal is to rejuvenate a depressed personality. Selling certain drugs aimed at improving mental health has been based, in part, on selling a condition. Examples are depression, obsessive-compulsive disorder, panic attacks, social anxiety disorder, sexual compulsion, and premenstrual dysphoria.[57] Some individuals may be affected by one or more of the disorders just mentioned, but it may not be serious enough to have a profound effect on their lives. But they reflect on their condition and convince themselves that they need medication to alleviate the problem. Thus they believe they will have "enhanced" themselves and their "playfulness" will return by starting on medication. Conditions such as extreme panic disorder or attention deficit hyperactivity disorder, if correctly diagnosed by a mental health professional, should come under control with appropriate medication, and a health professional should be the one to decide on the proper drug.

Prescription drug use has increased over a twelve-year period from 1999–2000 to 2012.[58] In 2012, fifty-nine percent of a sample population took some type of medication requiring a prescription. In adults sixty-five and older, thirty-nine percent reported taking multiple medications. The most frequently prescribed single drug in 2011–2012 was simvastatin, a drug used to lower cholesterol.[59] One reason why this particular statin emerged as number one was that it came off patent sooner than rival statins and was available at a lower price.

The overall amount spent on prescription drugs in 2014 was $374 billion, according to IMS Health, a medical industry marketing research firm.[60] To promote these health products, the pharmaceutical industry spent $4.8 billion on ads in 2014, an increase of thirty percent since 2011.[61] The greatest amount of advertising dollars ($3.2 billion) was spent on TV, followed by magazine ads ($1.2 billion), newspapers ($127 million), radio ($26 million), and billboards ($4 million).[62] With the advent of DTC advertising of prescription products, the promotion was directed at a broad population.[63] Drugs to lower cholesterol were among the most heavily advertised products, followed by antacids, antihistamines, antidepressants, and drugs for arthritis sufferers. These were medications that millions of consumers would find beneficial. Today, among the most heavily advertised products are Cialis and Viagra (erectile dysfunction), Xeljans, Humira, and Celebrex (all three for arthritis), Eliquis (blood clots), and Lyrica (fibromyalgia and painful diabetic neuropathy).[64] But there is now a trend to advertise expensive drugs aimed at a relatively small segment of the population. These drugs can cost $2000 to $12,000 a month. Thus, a relatively small number of patients "can make the expense of mass advertising worthwhile," according to Professor Timothy Calkins of Northwestern University.[65]

The American Medical Association has come out against DTCA.[66] They maintain that aggressive marketing could elevate prices and increase the demand for what for some patients are expensive and, in some cases, unnecessary drugs. Recently, Peter Bach wrote in the *New England Journal of Medicine* that "hand clapping for science is now inextricably linked to hand wringing over affordability ... the growth in spending on drugs has started to outstrip growth in other areas of health care."[67] The rate of introduction of new and presumably more expensive drugs has accelerated, with the FDA approval rate of new drugs increasing from "fifty-six to eighty-eight per cent in the past seven years." Assuming this will continue, this adds up to a "projected 13.6 percent increase from the last year to this year, as compared with a 5 percent growth in overall health spending." It seems obvious that somehow curtailing the stimulated desire of patients for the latest and most expensive drug would reduce the rate of health care spending.

New Zealand is the only other country that allows direct-to-consumer advertising of health care products requiring a prescription. Thus a New Zealander wishing to rejuvenate himself, to discover his real self, or stretch a few more years in the workplace, can determine which drug he might mention to his doctor in hopes of starting a new medication. How did this evolve? In 1981, the New Zealand Medicines Act did not consider the issue of advertising prescription drugs to the public. Recent articles in the *New Zealand Medical Journal* focused in the controversy of DTCA.[68] As in the U.S., advocates argue that the advertisements provide information to the patient, who is assumed to have at least some medical knowledge and make an informed choice about a medical product when he discusses the drug with his doctor. It is hoped a constructive dialogue will ensue.

Opponents of DTCA maintain that the information provided in the ads is "unbalanced," and is in favor of benefits over harm, leading to a demand for unnecessary prescriptions, increased costs, and possible iatrogenic harm.[69] As in the U.S., well-known personalities are often part of the positive image about the drug, leading to the impression on the part of the patient that the celebrity has researched the product or is a beneficiary of using the drug.[70] Opponents of DTCA also cite a study in New Zealand in which four out of five practicing general practitioners supported a ban on medical advertising to the public. Harm to the doctor-patient was cited as a reason.[71]

In New Zealand, a Pharmacology and Therapeutics Advisory Committee (PTAC) advises a Pharmaceutical Management Committee (PHARMAC) about which medicines should be listed in the New Zealand Pharmaceutical Schedule; that is, made available for treating the public.[72] In this scheme, PHARMAC has the final authority on funding. This has the effect of restricting the availability of new products and, presumably, of putting a brake on health-care costs. The pharmaceutical industry is critical of this restriction on the release of new products to doctors and their patients. Some products have been held up for years.[73] PTAC lists priorities for some products, but it is the impression of the pharmaceutical industry that there are instances in which there is a reprioritization of PTAC's recommendations carried out by PHARMAC. There have been instances in which products "with a lower PTAC priority have been funded ahead of those with a higher priority. Cost may well play a role in these decisions, but the lack of transparency makes it difficult to determine how or why priorities were determined."[74]

Between 2000 and 2009, Australia approved 136 new drugs to be listed in their Schedule of Pharmaceutical Benefits, while in New Zealand, only 59 were approved. The time taken for approval of new drugs was longer in New Zealand. The drugs listed in Australia but not New Zealand covered a wide range of therapeutic indications, some of which had "no alternative treatment in New Zealand."[75] Should the waiting list for new drugs in New Zealand be communicated to the public? It might stimulate greater interest in inquiring about new drug being evaluated. PHARMAC operates within a strictly capped budget. Only if the cap is lifted would there be more drugs approved.[76] A budget would have to have government approval, no easy task in view of rising drug prices.

Meanwhile, in the U.S., some action needs to be taken on the rapid rise of drug prices. This will require the cooperation of pharmaceutical firms, insurance companies, and health care professionals. Rejuvenation in the twenty-first century should not be so expensive.

Appendices

A. Daily Schedule of Station KFKB, Milford, Kansas. Hours of broadcast 5:30 a.m. to 8:00 p.m.

5:30 to 6:00 a.m. Health Lecture by announcer.
6:00 to 7:00 a.m. Bob Larkan and his Music Makers.
7:00 to 7:30 a.m. Hints to Good Health by announcer.
7:30 to 8:00 a.m. Bob Larkan and his Music Makers.
8:00 to 8:30 a.m. Professor Bert.
8:30 to 9:00 a.m. Old Time Entertainers.
9:00 to 9:30 a.m. Markets, weather, cash grain. Hauserman and Cook.
9:30 to 10:00 a.m. Medical Question Box. Dr. Brinkley.
10:00 to 11:00 a.m. Special features.
11:00 a.m. to 12:30 p.m. Steve Love and his Orchestra.
12:30 to 1:00 p.m. Health Talk by Dr. Brinkley.
1:00 to 2:00 p.m. Special features.
2:00 to 2:30 p.m. Dutch Hauserman and Cook.
2:30 to 3:00 p.m. Medical Question Box.
3:00 to 4:00 p.m. Bob Larkan and his Music Makers.
4:00 to 4:30 p.m. Uncle Sam and Dutch Hauserman.
4:30 to 5:45 p.m. Arthur Pizinger and his Orchestra.
5:45 to 6:00 p.m. Tell Me a Story Lady (for children).
6:00 to 6:15 p.m. Professor Bert, French language instruction.
6:15 to 6:30 p.m. Orchestra.
6:30 to 7:00 p.m. Dr. Brinkley.

There is nothing wrong about this schedule except that Brinkley overstepped the FRC rules by diagnosing and prescribing products from his pharmacy over the air. There was also considerable self-promotion.

Reference: Ansel Harlan Resler, "The Impact of John R. Brinkley on Broadcasting in the United States," PhD diss., Northwestern University, 1958, p. 317.

B. Excerpts from Stenographic Notes Taken of a Talk over XER Radio (broadcasting from Mexico) by Dr. John R. Brinkley on the Evening of November 8, 1933 (from enclosure No. 1 to Dispatch No. 46 from the American Consulate, Piedras Negras, Mexico, to the Secretary of State, Washington, D.C., Nov. 20, 1933).

Good-evening, everybody! You know your Cousin Paul would say, "This is Cousin Paul speaking. Well, I say, "This is your Uncle John speaking."

I am going to speak in connection with "Knowledge and Faith." Once I heard an old Negro preacher explain the difference between knowledge and faith. He said: "There is Brother Johnson sitting on the front seat with his wife and five children. His wife knows they are her children, that is knowledge; he believes they are his children, that is faith."

This is Dr. John R. Brinkley speaking from his home and hospital in Del Rio, Texas. I hope you are hearing what I have to say. I operated on Mr. Hill from Yuma, Arizona, and Mr. Bagly from Kansas this morning, and both are doing fine. Mrs. Hill is here with Mr. Hill.

I wish to announce that O.O. Robb has been sitting up all day. Alfred Nash sends greetings home. H.W. Walters of ... Kansas will go home tomorrow. James Ward is leaving for home tomorrow, Thursday.

No doubt you good people have seen an account of the death of Texas Guinan, the famous nightclub hostess, which took place in Vancouver, British Columbia. A pain struck her in the stomach and she had to leave the show and [go] into the hospital, where she was operated on and she did not recover. She suffered from colitis and she had been having trouble with her intestinal tract. Since Texas Guinan [died], I am glad that she died where Canadian doctors are honest enough to tell the truth as to the cause of her death. If she had died in this country, the doctors would have said she died of a ruptured appendix, because if they say colitis, that would be too much like what Dr. Brinkley has been telling you for years. I have been telling you for years that these aches and pains in the stomach are due to colitis. Not only grown people suffer from colitis; little boys and girls have colitis. Colitis is responsible for many of the pains you have. You will find mucus in the stool, bleeding and passing blood from children who suffer with colitis. You want to stay off of all starchy food, such as peas, potatoes, light bread, etc., as these starches form gas [in] the stomach. Colitis is a serious ailment if not treated in time, as it causes ulcers in the stomach, ulcers in the intestines. Now, I am not specializing in colitis, but you can control colitis by watching your diet and taking a mild laxative. The Del Rio Drug Store in Del Rio, Texas, sells colitis tablets which are a mild laxative ... and which are my personal prescription.

Nobody offers to cure colitis, but you can get relief for a long time by watching your diet and taking these colitis tablets. But the average woman will eat too much meat and too many eggs. Eat more vegetables and fruits. The trouble with most women [is] they do not eliminate sufficiently. You must eat more vegetables and fruits, fish, and lamb. What is better than a good lamb stew with nice carrots and onions? I got hungry myself after I had talked the other night about lamb stew and had Mrs. Brinkley's girl fix some for me and it was great. You will be greatly benefited by these colitis tablets which you can get from the Del Rio Drug Store at Del Rio, Texas. I want you to know that these tablets or any other medicine will not do you any good unless you have a lot of respect for your diet and I hope the death of Texas Guinan will not be in vain. I hope that this will call your attention to the fact that there is a lot of colitis. Do not gorge yourself but use common sense and you are going to get along a lot better.... I am requested by my friends, Mr. and Mrs. Elmer Boyer of Buenavista, Pennsylvania, to tell "hello" to them. These friends were listening for us and trying to hear, but it seems the giant station in Philadelphia interfered. On October 18 they heard very well and on October 28 they had some reception and this evening I hope Mr. and Mrs. Boyer are hearing me and if they do, I wish they would send a telegram at my expense. I would like to have their report. Mr. Elmer Boyer is one of our patients and Mr. Boyer is getting along fine and, if any of you would like to see some of our patients, look up Mr. Boyer. [Did these people know Brinkley was using their names?]

You people who are all the time grunting and groaning, never fit for anything, you are entirely to blame for your condition, whether it be financial or as to health; you have probably used poor judgment. I have been constantly been telling you for the last ten years that good health was something to guard and protect. Watch your health, guard it against colds.... Women should be doubly careful with their health, especially during the period of her change in life. Eat cooked fruits, cut out meats and eggs, but eat fish and lamb stew. A lamb stew with carrots, onions and other vegetables contains all the vitamins that are good for you women. Then you women who have these hot and cold flashes, get from the Del Rio Drug Store W.W. Capsules and constipation medicine and keep the old stream and glandular system clean. You will find ten thousand women have taken this advice and I receive thousands of letters and they tell me they have done this and you will do the same thing if you make up your mind, and remember if you are suffering from colitis the Del Rio Drug Store at Del Rio, Texas, has some tablets which will help you a great deal. [Note the frequent references to Brinkley's drug store in Del Rio.]

This radio talk and the following one were being monitored by the State Department in the U.S. in hope of encouraging the Mexican government to close Brinkley's radio station.

Reference: Resler, pp. 304–5.

C. Excerpts from Stenographic Notes Taken from a Talk over XER Radio by Dr. John R. Brinkley on the Evening of November 9, 1933 (from enclosure No. 2 to Dispatch No. 46 from the American Consulate, Piedras Negras, Mexico, to the Secretary of State, Washington, D.C., Nov. 20, 1933).

I am mighty glad to have a letter from Mr. and Mrs. Fred Springer of Manly, Iowa. They write, "We are fine and Fred is getting better every day. Dad is feeling better and has lost most of his shaking." We were surprised to hear that Dad Springer has

Appendices

lost most of his shaking as when we treated him we did not promise that he would lose this shaking.... In some of my talks I have told of some wonderful observations on things we do as a result of our prostate treatments. For instance, Mr. and Mrs. Springer's letter telling us that Dad Springer had lost his shaking after the prostate treatment, which we did not expect, but we often find results that we did not look for and our patients get rid of lots of things which we did not promise. For instance, Mr. Hill, who was operated on yesterday morning, has not for a long time been able to open his fingers or to work his toes and thought he had rheumatism and I claim there is no such thing as rheumatism, and today he is pointing out to Mrs. Hill and Mrs. Brinkley that he can work his fingers and work his toes, and results came to this man after twenty-four hours, which is astonishing and something that was not expected. So many good things happen top our cases that they are astounding.

Jacob Waldroll's brother and Mr. Stroll arrived on Wednesday and enjoyed Dr. Brinkley's treatment. Now you folks in Ohio who want to know what Dr. Brinkley can do, get in touch with Mr. Waldroll and Mr. Stroll.

Mr. and Mrs. J.T. Craeghen arrived with their son. Their son has been examined and accepted and will be operated on tomorrow. Mr. Harms was examined and accepted and I am going to operate on him tomorrow. We have quite a few cases which we have cured from Texas and in fact there are just a lot more patients coming from the state of Texas.

Before I forget it, I just heard from L.R. Brown that Mrs. Brown and baby girl are doing fine. You know I told you that they were the happy parents of a baby girl and glad to report that both father and mother are doing just fine and the baby is all right, too.

I have just received a nice letter from the Stonguise brothers. This letter was written by Karl. I have had the pleasure of treating both these brothers. They write that they received my photograph and say they are going to keep my photograph as long as they live, as they think I am the greatest man in the world. They say they boosted my work two years before I operated on them.

You folks in North Dakota and places where you are having sleet storms and where it is cold, you had better come to Del Rio, Texas, where the flowers are in bloom and everything is pretty and green. Mrs. John Foster just brought me a double rose, it is beautiful and I gave it to Johnny Boy and it is so beautiful that Johnny Boy has gone to bed with the rose. [No mention if the rose had thorns.]

J.A. Christopher of Seymour, Texas, writes me that this has been the best year he has had in twenty years, that he has been able to work 20 hours per day and if it had not been for the prostate operation he would not have been able to do this. He writes, "I think you are the greatest man on earth and do not see why they want to persecute you, but glad that you can practice in Texas. Thanks to you and Mrs. Brinkley."

G.H. Jones is feeling fine.... You folks who want to know about us in Texas can find out from G.H. Jones and J.A. Christopher. Mr. Christopher is a man 76 years old and was a mighty sick man when he came to me for prostate treatment. He was very much pleased with his operation, not only from a financial standpoint but he feels so much better. This man Christopher is sure a booster for me, well I am glad he is.

I have a letter from the Rev. John Wright of Idaho, and he writes, "I know you are getting settled in Del Rio, Texas, and that is the reason I have not heard from you.... I have another patient I will send you and will turn over the transportation certificate which you sent me." This makes 12 persons that he has sent to me for treatment.

C. Stenographic Notes—November 9, 1933

It is not unethical for doctors to get drunk, but it is unethical for me to practice. [It is not clear why Brinkley inserted this statement in his talk but there may have been rumors about his drinking when he left Kansas.]

Now that it is getting cold up there, ice and sleet, this is the time of year that that old prostate will give you trouble. Yes, I know it is hurting a lot. You are sitting there squirming around on that old cocklebur and yet you won't come and have that old prostate treated. You almost got persuaded to come and you hear about the weather and that sounds good to you and then there is an old devil comes into your mind that tells you that you are throwing your money away and then you hear me tell you that I will give you your money back if everything is not satisfactory and that there have been hundreds of cases cured and you go to your doctor and he tells you to stay away from prostate treatment and then you hear my offer to pay your expenses to Del Rio. Finally you may screw up a lot of nerve and after you have squirmed around on that old cocklebur you come and have an examination.

We are doing all we possibly can to make you come and be examined before it is too late. While we need your money and we need to have you come and see us, we are not going to accept your case unless we know we can cure you ... one knocker is worse than a thousand boosters. We are doing so much good for our patients. I told you about this man who was paralyzed, just like this gentleman whose fingers were stiff and his joints limbered up after the operation.

What more do you want, folks? I give you a guarantee on my work, then I offer to pay your railroad fare to and from Del Rio, I offer to do this work for you myself and offer to keep you in the Hotel Roswell, one of the most modern, best equipped hotels in the country, until you are perfectly able to leave. Mrs. Brinkley and I think there is nothing too good for our patients. We are offering you a first class station [situation?].

Then this lovely climate in Del Rio, where just a lot of lovely women, lovely men, and lovely children live, where the sun shines most of the time, and just think of that lovely mineral spring water from the San Felipe Spring. Just think of drinking that lovely spring water right out of the spring just as God gives it to you, and it does not cost you a cent. If you like to play golf we have a fine golf course, and if you get tired of golf and like to fish, you can go out to the river and catch all the bass. The bass are just jumping around in the river waiting to catch your bait, and there are catfish [weighing] 35–45 pounds. Or if you like to hunt we have wild turkeys, we have deer for you, and if you like to hunt big game we have on the other side of the river, at Villa Acuna, where the giant radio station is, mountain lions, and while there you can have one of the finest meals at Mrs. Crosby's of the Sabinas Café. You can get delicious Mexican food, all of them very clean, or this, that and the other thing. Those are some of the things you will enjoy here if you are thinking of coming down here to spend the winter. I do not know of any better place to go, and bless your heart, no one is going to charge you a penny if you are going to drink the fine San Felipe water.

If you come to Del Rio and stay through the winter and find you have to return home in the spring, before you go you can go to the Del Rio Drug Store and buy stomach tablets, colitis tablets, kidney medicine, women's capsules, cough medicines, anything you want, in fact, and get yourself cleaned out and cleaned up and you will be so well that you will feel like an entirely different individual when you leave this country. People are always coming here. On your way down here you can stop over in the lovely city of San Antonio, Texas, where there are so many interesting things to see and you will not want to pass up seeing that lovely place. Then you can go to Corpus Christi or to Galveston, to which you have a paved highway. Texas is really a kingdom all in itself, as it has all sorts of climate and every kind of vegetable. Texas is a good state to live in and a fine state (Resler, 307–9).

These two excerpts show how Brinkley used testimonials and the names of patients to further his practice. He certainly had no respect for the privacy of the patients by reading his report over the airways so anyone listening would know about Fred Springer's treatment. A few weeks after listening to Brinkley's broadcasts, the State Department Consul, who had been listening to Brinkley's radio programs, concluded that "he has an arresting and highly magnetic radio personality which radiates confidence, faith and sincerity." November 20, 1933 Resler, p. 246 (AMA archives 0097–11).

D. The Consulate in Piedras Negras continued their reporting on Brinkley in this description of his activities in Del Rio.

Dr. Brinkley has now leased the entire sixth floor of the Hotel Roswell in Del Rio, Texas, twelve to fifteen rooms, for his hospital and the entire basement for his X-ray room. He has opened a store on the ground floor which will sell his medicines. Advertisements for his treatments, which he has now been broadcasting over radio XER at Vila [sic] Acuna, Mexico, from his studio in Del Rio, Texas, describe principally his operation for reducing [the size] of the prostate gland. For the purpose of broadcasting he is reported to have leased some rooms in Del Rio over the J.C. Penny store ... where he broadcasts over his radio in Villa Acuna.

Doctor Brinkley has brought with him to Del Rio from Milford, Kansas, his nurses and two or three of his doctors, who have been working with him for several years. His office staff have not yet arrived in Del Rio, but it is reported that they are expected to arrive shortly. His caravan consisted of a number of truckloads of stuff from his studio and sanitarium.

The most prominent judge [in] Del Rio gave a very big reception and tea honoring Dr. and Mrs. Brinkley at his home on Saturday, November 4. It was attended by a great majority of the people of Del Rio. There is great enthusiasm in the town for him and apparently everyone is happy except for the [local] doctors. If his business grows as expected, he will probably lease, or purchase, the entire Roswell Hotel, which he doubtless could do at a relatively modest rental, since this big building of some eighty rooms is now reported to be running at considerable loss. It is expected that Dr. Brinkley's advent will gain population and business for Del Rio, and for Villa Acuna on the Mexican side. Dr. and Mrs. Brinkley have leased for their personal use one of the most beautiful homes in Del Rio, owned by Mr. Paul Edwards, and are now living there.

He is reported to have brought with him thirty families from Milford, who assisted him there and who will continue the work for him in Del Rio. It is reported that many houses in Del Rio, which had been vacant for some time for want of tenants, are now occupied by these families. The Del Rio public seems very happy over Dr. Brinkley's advent, which undoubtedly means more money and equipment.... As will be noted from the accompanying enclosures, he is taking care to broadcast the charms of Del Rio and the general locality over the world (Resler, p. 139.)

It seemed as though the financial gain to Del Rio, especially during the economic depression, overshadowed Brinkley's outrageous activities in Kansas.

E. Brinkley's accumulation of wealth is reflected in this description of him during a visit to Washington, D.C., to confer with former Vice-President Charles Curtis over his radio station.

Sparkling almost as much as Diamond Jim Brady in his palmiest days, Dr. John Brinkley of "goat gland fame," is here on his palatial yacht, modestly named Dr. Brinkley. If you don't think he sparkles—well, on his left hand is a diamond ring which weighs almost 13 karats. On his right hand is a diamond set fraternal ring. On his lapel twinkle two diamond-studded fraternal emblems. His cuff links also gleam. But his necktie is the masterpiece. There is a tie pin, set with a huge pear-shaped diamond, which appears to be at least six karats in size, surrounded with dozens of good-sized stones. And if that is not enough, the tie also holds a bar pin with a score or so of stones.

To complete the ensemble, from his heavy watch chain hangs another fraternal emblem, with more diamonds.

The doctor, whose goat gland work got him into a jam with the American Medical Association, and whose radio station got him into another jam with the Federal Communications Commission, is here to see his old friend Charley Curtis, former vice-president of the United States, and expects to sail tomorrow for the South on the 150 foot diesel-powered craft, one of the most luxurious yachts ever to come up the Potomac (Resler, p. 153, in the *Washington Times* August 26, 1935 [AMA archives 0096–08]).

Chapter Notes

Introduction

1. Eric Trimmer, *Rejuvenation: The Story of an Idea* (New York: A.S. Barnes, 1970), pp. 24–6.

2. Pankaj Kapahi and Jan Vig, "Aging—Lost in Translation?" *New England Journal of Medicine* 361 (2009): pp. 2669–70; S. Jay Olshansky, Leonard Hayflick, and Thomas Perls, "Anti-aging Medicine: The Hype and Reality—Part II," *Journal of Gerontology* 59A (2004): pp. 649–70; S. Mitchell Harman and Mark R. Blackman, "The Use of Growth Hormone for the Prevention of Treatment of the Effects of Aging," *Journal of Gerontology* 59A (2004): pp. 652–6; Carol Haber, "Anti-Aging: Why Now?" *Generations* 25 (4) (2001): pp. 9–14; Gerald J. Gruman, "The Rise and Fall of Prolongevity Hygiene," *Bulletin of the History of Medicine* 35 (1961): pp. 221–9.

3. Thomas R. Cole, *The Journey of Life: A Cultural History of Aging in America* (New York: Cambridge University Press, 1992), pp. 164–5, 172–5.

4. John Hill, *The Old Man's Guide to Health and Longer Life: With Rules for Diet, Exercise, and Physic*, 5th ed. (London: R. Baldwin and J. Ridley, 1764), pp. 4, 24.

5. Cole, pp. 164–7.

6. William Graebner, *A History of Retirement* (New Haven: Yale University Press, 1980), pp. 18–21.

7. Ibid.

8. William Osler, *Aequanimitas* (Philadelphia: Blakiston, 1947), pp. 31–2.

9. Ibid.

10. Ibid., p. 383.

11. Ibid.

12. Harvey Cushing, *The Life of Sir William Osler*, 2 vols. (Oxford: Clarendon Press, 1925), vol. 1, pp. 688–9.

13. Charles G. Roland, "The Infamous William Osler," *Journal of the American Medical Association* 193 (1985): pp. 436–8.

14. Michael Bliss, *William Osler: A Life in Medicine* (New York: Oxford University Press, 1999), pp. 324–5.

15. Osler, *Aequanimitas*, p. 383.

16. John F. Fulton, *Selected Readings in the History of Physiology*, 2nd ed. (Springfield, IL: Charles C. Thomas, 1966), pp. 414–7.

17. Christopher E. Forth, *Masculinity in the Modern West: Gender, Civilization and the Body* (New York: Palgrave Macmillan, 2008), pp. 169–70.

18. Chandak Sengoopta, "Rejuvenation and the Prolongation of Life: Science or Quackery?" *Perspectives in Biology and Medicine* 37 (1993): p. 65.

19. Franklin Martin, "Ovarian Transplantation," *Surgery, Gynecology & Obstetrics* 35 (1922): pp. 573–82; Hans H. Simmer, "Robert Tuttle Morris (1857–1943): A Pioneer in Ovarian Transplants," *Obstetrics and Gynecology* 35 (1970): pp. 314–26; Elizabeth Siegel Watkins, *The Estrogen Elixir* (Baltimore: Johns Hopkins University Press, 2007), pp. 12–13.

20. Anne Karpf, "The Liberation of Growing Older," *New York Times*, January 4, 2015.

Chapter 1

1. Charles Édouard Brown-Séquard, "The Effects on Man by Subcutaneous Injections of Liquid Obtained from Testicles of Animals," *Lancet* (July 20, 1889): pp. 105–7.

2. Ibid.

3. Christopher E. Forth, 99–100; Elizabeth Toon and Janet Golden, "Live Clean and Don't Go to Burlesque Shows: Charles Atlas as Health Advisor," *Journal of the History of Medicine 57* (2002): p. 57; Merriley Borell, "Brown-Séquard's Organotherapy," *Bulletin of the History of Medicine 50* (1976): pp. 309–20.

4. Arnold Adolph Berthold, "The Transplantation of the Testes," trans. D.F. Quiring, *Bulletin of the History of Medicine 16* (1944): pp. 399–401; Thomas R. Forbes, "A.A. Berthold and the First Endocrine Experiment: Some Speculation as to Its Origin," *Bulletin of the History of Medicine 23* (1949): pp. 263–7. The original article by Berthold was published in the *Archiv. fur Anatomie, Physiologie und Wissenschaftlich Medicine* (1849): pp. 42–6.

5. C.B. Jorgensin, "John Hunter, A.A. Berthold and the Origin of Endocrinology," *Acta historica scientiarum naturalium et medicinalium* 24 (1971): pp. 7–54(31); Thomas Schlich, *The Origin of Organ Transplantation* (Rochester: University of Rochester Press, 2010), p. 18.

6. John Hunter, *The Natural History of the Human Teeth: Explaining Their Structure, Use, Formation, Growth, and Disease* (London: J. Johnson, 1771), p. 4. Although the text deals primarily with teeth, Hunter included his research in testis transplantation.

7. Dr. W. Irvine to Professor Thomas Hamilton, London, June 17, 1771, in "John Hunter: Bicentenary Celebration," *Lancet* (February 18, 1928): pp. 359; Thomas R. Forbes, "Testes Transplantation Performed by John Hunter," *Endocrinology 41* (1947): pp. 329–30.

8. Editorial, "The Pentacle of Rejuvenescence," *British Medical Journal* 1 (June 22, 1889): p. 1416.

9. Roger E. Abrams, *The Dark Side of the Diamond* (Boston: Rounder Books, 2007), pp. 105–7; *Pittsburgh Commercial Gazette*, August 14, 1889.

10. Ibid., August 15, 1889.

11. Ibid., August 17, 1889.

12. Ibid., August 19, 1889.

13. Baseballhalloffame.org.

14. William A. Hammond, "Experiments Relative to the Therapeutic Value of the Expressed Juice of the Testicles When Hypodermically Introduced into the Human System," *New York Medical Journal* 50 (1889): pp. 232–4.

15. Ibid., p. 233.

16. Ibid.

17. Ibid., p. 234.

18. Ibid.

19. Editorial, "Is There an Elixir of Life?" *Boston Medical and Surgical Journal* 121 (August 15, 1889): pp. 167–8.

20. New York Correspondent, *Lancet* 1 (January 4, 1890): pp. 57–8.

21. Ibid.

22. Charles Édouard Brown-Séquard, "On a New Therapeutic Method Consisting in the Use of Organic Liquids Extracted from Glands and Other Organs," *British Medical Journal* (June 3, 10, 1893): pp. 1145–7, 1212–4.

23. J.M.D. Olmsted, *Charles Édouard Brown-Séquard, A Nineteenth Century Neurologist and Endocrinologist* (Baltimore: Johns Hopkins University Press, 1946), p. 232.

24. Obituary, *Lancet* (April 7, 1894): pp. 876, 975; *New York Times*, April 3, 1894.

25. Michael J. Aminoff, *Brown-Séquard: A Visionary of Science* (New York: Raven Press, 1993), p. 171.

26. George R. Murray, "Note on the Treatment of Myxoedema by Hypodermic Injection of an Extract of the Thyroid Gland of a Sheep," *British Medical Journal* 2 (October 10, 1891): pp. 796–7.

27. George R. Murray, "The Life-History of the First Case of Myxoedema Treated with Thyroid Extract," *British Medical Journal* 1 (March 15, 1920): pp. 359–60.

28. George Oliver and Edward Sharpey-Schafer, "On the Physiologic Action of Extract of the Suprarenal Capsule," *Journal of Physiology (London) Proceedings* 16 (1894): pp. i–iv; George Oliver and Edward Sharpey-Schafer, *Journal of Physiology (London)* 18 (1895): pp. 230–76. The other important secretion from the adrenal gland is cortisone, which was isolated in 1936 by Edward Kendall.

29. Ernest Henry Starling, "The Chemical Correlations of the Function of the Human Body," *Lancet* (August 5, 1905): pp. 321–4.

30. Alexander Wood, "Treatment of Neuralgic Pains by Narcotic Injections," *British Medical Journal* 2 (1858): pp. 721–3; Norman Howard-Jones, "A Critical Study of the Origins and Early Development of the Hypodermic Medication," *Journal of the History of Medicine and Allied Sciences* 2 (1947): pp. 201–49.

31. Joseph Lister, "The Antiseptic Prin-

ciple in the Practice of Surgery," *British Journal of Surgery* 2 (1867): p. 246.

32. Michael Bliss, *The Discovery of Insulin*, 25th anniversary ed. (Chicago: University of Chicago Press, 2007), p. 26.

33. Merrily Borell, pp. 309–20; Theodore B. Schwartz, "Henry Harrower and the Turbulent Beginning of Endocrinology," *Annals of Internal Medicine* 131 (1999): pp. 702–6.

34. Lewellys F. Barker, "The Study of the Internal Secretions: An Introduction," *Endocrinology* 1 (1917): pp. 1–4.

35. Walter B. Cannon, "Roy Haskins: An Appreciation," *Endocrinology* 30 (1942): pp. 843–5.

36. F.M. Pottenger, "The Association for the Study of Internal Secretions. Its Past: Its Future," *Endocrinology* 30 (1942): p. 846.

Chapter 2

1. *Quarterly Bulletin, Northwestern University Medical School* 21 (1947): p. 92.

2. Victor D. Lespinasse, "Transplantation of the Testicle," *Journal of the American Medical Association* 61 (1913): pp. 1869–70.

3. Alexis Carrel, "Nobel Lecture, Suture of Blood-vessels and Transplantation of Organs," (December 11, 1912), http://Nobel prize.org.

4. Lespinasse, "Transplantation of the Testicle," p. 1869.

5. Ibid., p. 1870.

6. Levi J. Hammond and Howard A. Sutton, "An Abstract Report of a Case of Transplantation of a Testicle," *International Clinics* 22 (1912): pp. 150–55.

7. Ibid., p. 1970.

8. Susan E. Lederer, *Flesh and Blood: Organ Transplantation and Blood Transfusion in Twentieth Century America* (New York: Oxford University Press, 2008), p. 23.

9. Victor D. Lespinasse, "Transplantation of the Testicle," *The Chicago Medical Recorder* 36 (1914): pp. 401–3.

10. Ibid., p. 402.

11. Victor D. Lespinasse, *Impotency: Its Treatment by Transplantation of the Testicle*, Surgical Clinics of Chicago (Philadelphia: W.B. Saunders, 1918), pp. 281–8; *The Social Evil in Chicago* (Chicago: The Vice Commission of Chicago, Gunthorp-Warren Printing, 1911). Perhaps the heated sexual atmosphere surrounding houses of prostitution in Chicago led to a desire to capture waning libido. The annual profit from prostitution at this time was estimated at over fifteen million dollars (p. 113).

12. Lespinasse, p. 282.

13. Ibid., p. 288.

14. "McCormick's Surgeon Silent on Gland Story," *Chicago Daily Tribune*, June 18, 1922.

15. Emmett Dedmon, *Fabulous Chicago* (New York: Random House, 1953), pp. 310–16.

16. Robert J. Casey, *More Interesting People* (New York: Bobbs-Merrell, 1947), pp. 20–24. The author points out that this story "marked an end to any Victorian reticence that might have been left in the newspaper business by printing detailed reports of ... Harold McCormick's gland operation."

17. Ibid., pp. 22–3.

18. "McCormick Out in Short Time," *Chicago Daily Tribune*, June 20, 1922.

19. Ibid. This article added that the donor has been amply rewarded and is "long gone."

20. "Gland Grafting Held to Benefit Women Also," *Chicago Daily Tribune*, June 22, 1922. In addition to documenting Dr. Lespinasse's activities, the health editor of the *Tribune*, Dr. W.A. Evans, stated gland surgery in women has "not been attended with the same success as in the case of men." Apparently, Dr. Evans was impressed with the success of gland surgery in men.

21. "No Human Gland in Operation on H.F. McCormick," *Chicago Daily Tribune*, June 24, 1922.

22. Dedmon, *Fabulous Chicago*, p. 314.

23. "H.F. McCormick to Sue for Libel," *Chicago Daily Tribune*, June 29, 1922.

24. Dedmon, *Fabulous Chicago*, pp. 314–6.

25. Ibid., p. 316.

26. "Parts," *Time*, August 24, 1925, p. 26.

27. Victor D. Lespinasse, "Obstructive Sterility in the Male," *Journal of the American Medical Association* 70 (1918): pp. 448–50.

28. Victor D. Lespinasse, "Sterility in the Male," *Surgery, Gynecology & Obstetrics* 24 (1917): pp. 597–9.

29. Victor D. Lespinasse, "Sterility Studies," *Journal of the American Medical Association* 68 (1917): pp. 345–8.

30. Victor D. Lespinasse, "Abstract of Discussion on Papers of Drs. Meaker,

Hotchkiss and Hagner," *Journal of the American Medical Association* 107 (1936): p. 1854.

31. Loyal Davis, *Neurological Surgery* (Philadelphia: Lea & Febiger, 1936), p. 405.

32. Alan R. Cohen and Axel Perneczky, "Endoscopy and the Management of Third Ventricular Lesions," in *Surgery of the Third Ventricle,* edited by Michael L.J. Apuzzo (Baltimore: Williams & Wilkins, 1998), pp. 889–91.

33. Victor D. Lespinasse, Discussion, August A. Werner paper, "The Male Climacteric," *Journal of the American Medical Association* 132 (1946): p. 194.

34. "Deaths," *Journal of the American Medical Association* 132 (1946): p. 1102.

35. Vincent J. O'Conor, "Appreciation," *Quarterly Bulletin, Northwestern University Medical School* 21 (Spring 1947): p. 92.

36. "Obituary, Dr. V.D. Lespinasse," *New York Times,* December 16, 1946.

37. Yelfin R. Sheykin, Alex Mishail, and David Schulsinger, "Andrology Evolution: Life and Works of Victor Lespinasse," *Journal of Urology* 179 (supplement 2008): pp. 307–8.

38. Chicago Wesley Memorial Hospital Archives (now Northwestern Memorial), December 20, 1947.

Chapter 3

1. William K. Beatty, "G. Frank Lydston—Urologist, Author and Pioneer Transplanter," *Proceedings of the Institute of Medicine Chicago* 43 (1990): p. 35.

2. Ibid., p. 36.

3. Ibid.

4. G. Frank Lydston, *The Surgical Diseases of the Genito-Urinary Tract: Venereal and Sexual Disease: A Text-Book for Students and Practitioners* (Philadelphia: F.A. Davis, 1889).

5. G. Frank Lydston, "Implantation of the Generative Glands and its Therapeutic Possibilities," *New York Medical Journal* 100 (1914): pp. 745–6.

6. Ibid. In 1920, Lydston revealed that the testicle was placed outside his office window to preserve it in a cold environment: *Southern California Practitioner* 35 (1920): p. 57.

7. Lydston, "Implantation of the Generative Glands," pp. 752–3.

8. Ibid., p. 818.

9. Ibid., p. 753.

10. Ibid., p. 818.

11. Robert Tuttle Morris, "Heterografting of Testicle," *New York Medical Journal* 100: (1917): pp. 753–4, 819.

12. Lydston, p. 819.

13. Ibid. pp. 862–9.

14. Ibid., pp. 864–6.

15. Ibid.

16. Ibid., p. 869.

17. Ibid.

18. Ibid. pp., 914–7.

19. G. Frank Lydston, "Experiments with Emulsions of Organs Taken from the Dead Human Body and Sex Glands of the Lower Animals," *American Medicine* 20 (1914): pp. 767–73.

20. Ibid., p. 769.

21. Ibid.

22. Ibid., p. 772.

23. Ibid.

24. Ibid.

25. G. Frank Lydston, "Sex Gland Implantation," *Journal of the American Medical Association* 66 (1916): pp. 1540–3.

26. Ibid., p. 1542.

27. Ibid.

28. Ibid.

29. G. Frank Lydston, *Impotence and Sterility with Aberrations of the Sexual Function and Sex Gland Implantation* (Chicago: Riverton Press, 1917), pp. 142–6.

30. Ibid., p. 143.

31. Ibid., 146.

32. Ibid., p. 228.

33. Max Thorek, *A Surgeon's World* (Philadelphia: Lippincott, 1924), pp. 180–91.

34. Morris Fishbein, *An Autobiography* (Garden City, NY: Doubleday, 1969), p. 36.

35. *Chicago Urological Society Minutes,* vol. 2, November 15, 1917.

36. G. Frank Lydston, "Cases Showing Remote Results of Testicular Implantation," *Journal of the American Medical Association* 70 (1918): pp. 907–8.

37. Ibid.

38. G. Frank Lydston, "Two Remarkable Cases of Testicular Implantation," *New York Medical Journal* 113 (1921): pp. 232–3.

39. "America Was First in Grafting," *New York Times,* August 15, 1920, p. 8.

40. G. Frank Lydston, "The Flies on the Chariot Wheel," *Illinois State Medical Journal* 42 (1922): pp. 97–101.

41. Deaths, "George Frank Lydston,"

Journal of the American Medical Association 80 (1923): p. 787.

42. Beatty, p. 63.

43. Ibid., p. 35.

44. H. Lyons Hunt, "Further Experiences in Gland Transplantation," *New York State Journal of Medicine* 23 (1923): p. 448.

45. H. Lyons Hunt, "Experiences in Testicle Transplantation," *Endocrinology* 6 (1922): pp. 652–4.

46. Ibid., p. 652.

47. Ibid., p. 653.

48. Hunt, "Further Experiences in Gland Transplantation," p. 448.

49. Ibid., p. 490.

50. Ibid.

51. Ibid., p. 491.

52. H. Lyons Hunt, "New Theory of the Function of the Prostate Deduced from Gland Transplantation in Physicians," *Endocrinology* 9 (1925): pp. 479–89.

53. Ibid., pp. 483–4.

54. Ibid., pp. 484–8. The technique to remove the prostate was not specified. However, after prostate surgery, sexual function may return after a certain period of time. Hunt, not being a urologist, may not have known this fact. Therefore, had no transplant been done, the end result might have been the same.

55. Lawrence K. Altman, *Who Goes First? The History of Self-Experimentation in Medicine* (New York: Random House, 1987), pp. 45–51.

56. Ibid.

57. *New York Times*, "Pennsylvania Surgeon Operates on Himself," February 16, 1921.

58. *New York Times*, "Operates on Himself for the Second Time," February 16, 1932.

59. *New York Times*, April 2, 1933.

Chapter 4

1. Leo L. Stanley, *Men at Their Worst* (New York: Appleton-Century, 1940), p. 42; Leo Stanley, "Twenty Years at San Quentin," Stanley Papers, California State Historical society, MS 2061, pp. 1–8.

2. Stanley, *Men at Their Worst*, pp. 40, 283–4.

3. Herbert M. Evans to L.L. Stanley, July 12, 1916, Leo Stanley Papers, Lane Medical Archives, Lane Medical Library, Stanford University School of Medicine,

MSS 15, 66.1. Evans would later gain fame for discovering vitamin E.

4. Walter C. Alvarez, "Difference in the Latent Period and Form of the Contraction Curve in the Muscle Strips from Different Parts of the Mammalian Stomach," *American Journal of Physiology* 42 (1917): pp. 435–49.

5. Howard C. Naffziger to L.L. Stanley, February 19, 1923, Leo Stanley Papers, Lane Medical Archives, Lane Medical Library, Stanford University School of Medicine, MSS 15.

6. Stanley, *Men at Their Worst*, pp. 3–6.

7. Ibid., p. 6.

8. G. Frank Lydston, "Implantation of the Generative Glands and Its Therapeutic Possibilities," *New York Medical Journal* 199 (October 14, 1914): pp. 745–53.

9. Stanley, *Men at their Worst*, pp. 62; "Twenty Years at San Quentin," p. 13.

10. G. Frank Lydston, "Further Observation on Sex Gland Implantation," *Journal of the American Medical Association* 72 (1919): p. 398.

11. Leo Stanley, "Experiences in Testicle Transplantation," *California State Journal of Medicine* 18 (1920): pp. 251–3.

12. Lydston, (1919): p. 398.

13. L.L. Stanley and G. David Kelker, "Testicle Transplantation," *Journal of the American Medical Association* 74 (1920): pp. 1501–3.

14. Ibid., p. 1502.

15. Ibid.

16. Ibid.

17. Stanley, "Experiences in Testicle Transplantation," pp. 251–3. This paper omitted the case of a seventy-two-year-old convict in jail for "lascivious behavior" with a minor. Might there have been some criticism for transplanting a testicle into this man?

18. Ibid., p. 253.

19. Ibid.

20. L.L. Stanley, "An Analysis of One Thousand Testicular Substance Implantations," *Endocrinology* 6 (1922): pp. 787–94.

21. Ibid., pp. 788–9.

22. Ibid., p. 790.

23. Ibid., p. 789.

24. Ibid.

25. George Henderson, *Oakland Tribune*, cited in L.L. Stanley, "News Men I Have Known," California Historical Society, Leo Stanley Papers, MS 13031.

26. Stanley, "An Analysis of One Thou-

sand Testicular Substance Implantations,"
p. 788.

27. Ibid., p. 790.

28. Ibid., p. 794.

29. G. Frank Lydston to L.L. Stanley, March 2, 1923, Leo Stanley Papers MSS 15, 66.1 Lane Medical Archives.

30. Robert Day to L.L. Stanley, November 12, 1921, Leo Stanley Papers MSS 15, 66.1, Lane Medical Archives; Patrick M. McGrady, Jr., *The Youth Doctors* (New York: Coward-McCann, 1968), pp. 48–9.

31. L.L. Stanley to Kiwanis Club, San Francisco, January 17, 1921, Leo Stanley Papers MSS 15. 66.1.

32. Stanley, "An Analysis of One Thousand Testicular Substance Implantations," p. 787.

33. Roy G. Hoskins, "Some Recent Work on Internal Secretions," *Endocrinology* 6 (1922): p. 621.

34. Stanley, *Men at Their Worst*, p. 113.

35. L.L. Stanley, "The Effects of Testicular Implantations on Glycosuria," *Endocrinology* 11 (1927): pp. 305–12.

36. Stanley, *Men at Their Worst*, pp. 93–9; Stanley, "News Men I Have Known," pp. 3–4.

37. Stanley, *Men at Their Worst*, p. 95.

38. Ibid., p. 96.

39. Ibid.

40. Leo Leonidas Stanley, "The Buck Kelly Case," *The American Journal of Medical Jurisprudence* 2 (1939): pp. 45–52.; Leo L. Stanley, *My Most Unforgettable Convicts* (Winnipeg: Greywood Publishing, 1967), pp. 116–7.

41. Stanley, "News Men I Have Known," pp. 3–4.

42. Stanley, *Men at Their Worst*, p. 97.

43. Ibid., p. 98.

44. Ibid., p. 99.

45. Stanley, "The Buck Kelly Case," pp. 45–52.

46. Stanley, "News Men I Have Known," p. 6.

47. "Attributes All Crime to Glands," *New York Times*, February 9, 1930.

48. "Criminal Glands," *Time*, February 17, 1930.

49. Leo L. Stanley, "Voluntary Sterilization in Prison," *Medical Record* (March 18, 1936): pp. 1–5.

50. Ibid.

51. Leo L. Stanley, interview with Carla Ehat and Anne Kent, August 7, 1974, transcript, Oral History Project of Marin County Free Library, San Rafael, California.

52. Ibid.

53. Bernice Freeman, "San Quentin's 'Chief Croaker,' Dr. Leo Stanley to Retire April 1st," *San Francisco Chronicle*, February 26, 1951.

54. Leo Stanley Interview, Marin County Free Library.

55. Stanley, "News Men I Have Known," pp. 29, 42.

56. Ibid.

57. Ibid.

58. Deaths, "Dr. Leo Stanley," *San Francisco Examiner*, November 16, 1976.

59. Bernice Freeman, "San Quentin's Chief Croaker," *San Francisco Chronicle*, February 26, 1951.

60. Ibid.

61. L.L. Stanley, "Nasal Fracture," *Surgery, Gynecology & Obstetrics* 27 (1918): pp. 609–11.

62. Josiah D. Rich, Sarah E. Wakerman, and Samuel L. Dickman, "Medicine and the Epidemic of Incarceration in the United States," *New England Journal of Medicine* 364 (2011): pp. 2081–3.

Chapter 5

1. Serge Voronoff, *Rejuvenating by Grafting*, trans. Fred Imianitoff (London: George Allen & Unwin, 1925), pp. 57–60.

2. Ibid., pp. 60–7.

3. Ibid., pp. 68–70.

4. David Hamilton, *The Monkey Gland Affair* (London: Catto & Windus, 1986), pp. 1–2.

5. Ibid., p. 2.

6. Alexis Carrel, "Nobel Lecture," Nobel Prize.org/medicine/laureates/1912/carrel-lecture.html.

7. Serge Voronoff to Alexis Carrel, March 7, 1913, Carrel Papers, Special Collections Research Center, Georgetown University Library, box 42, sec. 14–3, folder 49; Hamilton, pp. 5–6.

8. Serge Voronoff to Alexis Carrel.

9. Hamilton, p. 11.

10. Serge Voronoff, *Life: A Study of the Means of Restoring Vital Energy and Prolonging Life* (New York: E.P. Dutton, 1920), p. 71.

11. Hamilton, pp. 20–1.

12. Ibid.

13. Ibid., pp. 21–2.

14. Ibid.

15. Ibid., p. 23.

16. Ibid., pp. 31–3.

17. Ibid., p. 32.

18. Ibid., p. 33.

19. Max Thorek, *A Surgeon's World* (Philadelphia: J.B. Lippincott, 1943), pp. 182–4.

20. Hamilton, pp. 41–2.

21. Voronoff, *Life*, p. xix.

22. Ibid., p. 8. Here Voronoff places more emphasis on longevity rather than just rejuvenation.

23. Ibid., pp. 112–3.

24. Beatrice Hahn, "Research Summary," http://www.upenn.edu/micro/faculty/hahn.html. Voronoff was disappointed the monkeys did not thrive in his monkey colony; some died on the trip to the breeding colony. They may have been infected with the virus. Hamilton, p. 91.

25. Voronoff, *Life*, pp. 146–7.

26. Book review, Serge Voronoff, *Greff Testiculaires* (Paris: G. Doin, 1922): p. 763.

27. "Voronoff Hooted by French Doctors," *New York Times*, October 6, 1922.

28. "Voronoff Patient Tells of New Life," *New York Times*, October 7, 1922. Voronoff brought a "rejuvenated" patient to this meeting as a demonstration of his success; the man died a year later, on August 21, 1923 (*New York Times*).

29. Book review, Serge Voronoff, *Greff Testiculaires*, *Lancet* 1 (November 18, 1922): pp. 1079–80.

30. Book review, Édouard Retterer and Serge Voronoff, *La Grande Génitale Male et Les Glandes Endocrines* (Paris: Librarie Octave Doin, 1921); Book review, *Endocrinology* 5 (1921): p. 777.

31. *New York Times*, October 6, 1922.

32. "America Was First in Gland Grafting," *New York Times*, August 15, 1920.

33. Moyer S. Fleisher and Leo Loeb, "The Relative Importance of Stroma and Parenchyma in the Growth of Certain Organs in Culture Media," *Proceedings of the Society of Experimental Biology and Medicine* 8 (1911): pp. 133–8; Leo Loeb, "Growth of Tissues in Culture Media and its Significance for the Analysis of Growth Phenomena," *Anatomical Record* 6 (1912): pp. 109–120.

34. "Obituary, Mme. Frances E.B. Voronoff," *New York Times*, March 6, 1921.

35. "Voronoff Buys Monkeys," *New York Times*, November 18, 1922.

36. "Two Monkeys Flee," *New York Times*, August 1, 1923.

37. "Voronoff to Establish Monkey Farm Near Nice," *New York Times*, December 23, 1925.

38. Dorothy Sayers, *The Unpleasantness at the Bellona Club* (London: Victor Gollancz, 1972), pp. 181–2. The book was originally published in 1928.

39. Arthur Conan Doyle, "The Adventures of the Creeping Man," in *Sherlock Holmes: The Complete Novels and Stories*, vol. 2 (New York: Bantam Classic, 2003), pp. 652–73.

40. Voronoff, *Rejuvenation by Grafting*, pp. 68–127.

41. Ibid., pp. 118–9.

42. "Voronoff Now Plans Super-Race of Sheep," *New York Times*, July 1923.

43. "Voronoff Operates on French Race Horse," *New York Times*, October 27, 1923.

44. "Horse Balks Voronoff," *New York Times*, December 5, 1923.

45. A. Eichhorn, "Recent Developments in Rejuvenation by Transplantation of Internal Secretory Tissues," *Veterinary Medicine* 20 (1925): pp. 291–5.

46. Foreign Letters, "Voronoff's Conclusions on Testicular Grafting Questioned," *Journal of the American Medical Association* 90 (1928): p. 1489.

47. Editorial. "The Voronoff Operation in Stock-Breeding," *Nature* 121 (May 5, 1928): pp. 717–8.

48. Hamilton, pp. 125–7.

49. Ibid., p. 126.

50. Ibid., p. 127.

51. Ibid., p. 128.

52. "Gland Transplantation Reported a Failure," *New York Times*, January 3, 1928.

53. "Wife Sues Voronoff," *New York Times*, February 26, 1928.

54. Navarre Atkinson, "Tells New Method of Rejuvenation," *New York Times*, January 24, 1928.

55. "Rejuvenation Row Rends the Viennese," *New York Times*, February 5, 1928.

56. "Voronoff Foresees 150 Years of Life," *New York Times*, May 24, 1928.

57. Ibid.

58. "Condemns Gland Grafting," *New York Times*, June 15, 1928.

59. "Inge Assails Voronoff," *New York Times*, June 4, 1928.

60. George Bernard Shaw, Letter to the Editor, *Daily News (London)*, in *The Saturday Review of Literature* (July 14, 1928): p. 1043. The letter was reprinted in its

entirety in the *Saturday Review.*

61. "Tells of Gains Made in the Fight on Old Age," *New York Times,* August 24, 1929.

62. Ibid. The discovery of testosterone was by a German chemist, Adolf Butenandt, and a Swiss chemist, Leopold Ruzicka.

63. Serge Voronoff and George Alexandrescu, *Testicular Grafting from Ape to Man,* trans. Theodore C. Merrill (London: Brentano's, 1929), pp. 113–6.

64. Ibid., p. 27.

65. Ibid., pp. 27–8.

66. Ibid., p. 28.

67. Eunice Fuller Barnard, "Our Quest for the Fountain of Youth," *New York Times,* November 16, 1930.

68. Alexis Carrel, "Physiological Time," *Science* 74 (1931): pp. 618–21; "Carrel Is Dubious on Rejuvenation," *New York Times,* December 22, 1931.

69. "Voronoff, 64, Weds Viennese, Age 20," *New York Times,* April 28, 1934.

70. Serge Voronoff, *Sidelights from the Surgery: Human Experience in the Consulting Room* (London: Pallas, 1939), pp. 18–22.

71. "Voronoff Corrects His Critics," *New York Times,* August 25, 1940.

72. Hamilton, 141; "Dr. Serge Voronov Surgeon, 85, Dead," *New York Times,* September 4, 1951. The spelling of his name was corrected in the following article in the *Times.*

73. "Voronoff Buried Secretly," *New York Times,* September 12, 1951.

74. "Obituary, Dr. Serge Voronoff," *The Times (London),* September 3, 1951.

75. Max Thorek, *The Human Testis* (Philadelphia: J.B. Lippincott, 1924), pp. 397–400.

76. Ibid., p. 443.

77. Ibid.

78. Ibid., p. 444.

79. Thorek, *A Surgeon's World* (Philadelphia: Lippincott, 1943), p. 190.

80. Ibid.

81. Ibid., p. 188.

82. Kenneth M. Walker, "Testicular Grafts," *Lancet* 1 (February 16, 1924): pp. 319–326.

83. Ibid., p. 321.

84. Ibid., p. 323–4.

85. Ibid., p. 324–5.

86. Martha Feldman, *The Castrato* (Oakland: University of California Press, 2015), p. xi.

87. Ibid., p. xii.

88. Ibid., p. 5.

89. Ibid., p. 62.

90. Ibid., p. 80.

91. Ibid., p. xvii.

92. Ibid., pp. xvii, 70.

Chapter 6

1. Eugene Steinach, *Sex and Life* (New York: Viking, 1940), pp. 138–9. Steinach had previously performed testicle transplants in animals, and later encouraged urologists in Vienna to perform transplants in humans.

2. Ibid., pp. 132–8. Steinach uses the words reactivation, revitalization, and rejuvenation in the same context.

3. Ibid., pp. 166–7.

4. Ibid., p. 176.

5. Ibid., pp. 179–89.

6. Ibid.

7. Ibid., p. 180.

8. Ibid., pp. 180–1.

9. Ibid.

10. George Corners (George Sylvester Viereck), *Rejuvenation: How Steinach Makes People Young* (New York: Thomas Seltzer, 1923), pp. 57–63. Corners interviewed Peter Schmidt, a German urologist, and a number of his patients, who believed the operation had rejuvenated them.

11. Steinach, p. 184.

12. Harry Benjamin, "Preliminary Communication Regarding Steinach's Method of Rejuvenation," *New York Medical Journal* 114 (1921): pp. 687–92; "Theory and Practice of the Steinach Operation," *New York Medical Journal* 116 (1922): pp. 203–7.

13. Harry Benjamin, "The Steinach Operation: Report of 22 Cases with Endocrine Interpretation," *Endocrinology* 6 (1922): pp. 776–86. The "interpretation" referred to in the title was a clinical impression, not a laboratory analysis.

14. Harry Benjamin, "The Steinach Method Applied to Women," *New York Medical Journal* 118 (1923): pp. 750–3.

15. Ibid., p. 751.

16. Ibid., p. 753.

17. Emily Wortis Leider, *California's Daughter: Gertrude Atherton and Her Times* (Stanford: Stanford University Press, 1991), pp. 291–2.

18. Ibid., p. 30–3.

19. Ibid., p. 305.

20. Ibid., p. 307.

21. Sharon Romm, *The Unwelcome Intruder: Freud's Struggle with Cancer* (New York: Praeger, 1983), pp. 17–23.

22. Ibid., pp. 23, 83–4.

23. Ibid., p. 139.

24. Current Comment, "Glandular Therapy," *Journal of the American Medical Association* 83 (1924): p. 1004.

25. Robert Oslund, "Vasectomy on Dogs," *American Journal of Physiology* 70 (1924): pp. 111–7.

26. Carl Moore and Robert Oslund, "Experiments on the Sheep Testis—Cryptorchidism, Vasectomy and Scrotal Insulation," *American Journal of Physiology* 67 (1924): pp. 495–508.

27. Robert Oslund, "The Behavior of the Testis in Transplantation, Experimental Cryptorchidism, Vasectomy, Scrotal Insulation, and Heat Application," *Endocrinology* 8 (1924): pp. 422–42.

28. Carl Moore, "The Behavior of the Testis in Transplantation, Experimental Cryptorchidism, Vasectomy, Scrotal Insulation, and Heat Application," *Endocrinology* 8 (1924): pp. 495–508.

29. Carl Moore, "On the Physiological Properties of the Gonads as Controllers of Somatic and Psychical Characteristics. II. Growth of Gonadectomized Male and Female Rats," *Journal of Experimental Zoology* 28 (1919): pp. 459–67.

30. Maxim Bing, "The First World Sex Congress," *Science (supplement)* 64 (1926): p. xii.

31. Adolph Granat, "Eugene Steinach's Work on Rejuvenation," *New York Medical Journal* 112 (1920): pp. 612–3.

32. Corners, *Rejuvenation*, p. 4.

33. Robert Fitzroy Foster, *W.B. Yeats: A Life*, vol. 2: *The Arch Poet 1915–39* (Oxford: Oxford University Press, 2003), p. 496.

34. Ibid., p. 499.

35. Stephen Lock, "'O that I Were Young Again': Yeats and the Steinach Operation," *British Medical Journal* 287 (1983): pp. 1964–8; Foster, p. 504–5.

36. Foster, pp. 510–11.

37. Ibid., p. 512.

38. "William Butler Yeats Biography," Famous Poets and Poems.com.

39. Steinach, p. 129.

40. Ibid., p. 82.

41. Steinach, pp. 24–6.

42. Harry Benjamin, Letter to the Editor, *New York Times*, June 2, 1944.

43. Leider, p. 307.

Chapter 7

1. R. Alton Lee, *The Bizarre Careers of John R. Brinkley* (Lexington: University Press of Kentucky, 2002), pp. 29–30; Gerald Carson, *The Roguish World of Doctor Brinkley* (New York: Holt Rinehart and Winston, 1960), p. 32. Of these two biographies, Lee's is the more complete and well documented.

2. Office of the Surgeon General to Arthur Cramp, Archives, American Medical Association, 0096–04.

3. Lee, p. 2.

4. Carson, pp. 16–7.

5. Lee, pp. 12–3. Sally was twenty-two, John a year younger. He stood five feet, six inches.

6. Carson, p. 17. This exposure to what amounted to quackery would play a role in Brinkley's future.

7. Winston U. Solberg, *Reforming Medical Education* (Urbana: University of Illinois Press, 2009), p. 154.

8. Lee, p. 16.

9. Ibid., p. 17.

10. Ibid., p. 20.

11. Richard Harrison Shyrock, *Medical Licensing in America, 1650–1965* (Baltimore: Johns Hopkins University Press, 1967), pp. 60–3; Carl F. Ameringer, *State Medical Boards and the Politics of Public Protection* (Baltimore: Johns Hopkins University Press, 1999), pp. 19–20; Erika Janik, *Marketplace of the Marvelous* (Boston: Beacon Press, 2014), pp. 16, 61, 254. During the early 19th century, medical licensing was thwarted by the rise of populist political movements, which were anti-elitist and sought to use common sense and personal experience as criteria for the practice of medicine.

12. Carson, p. 25; Lee, p. 22. Lee points out that graduates from the Kansas City School were required to pay $500 to take the Missouri State Medical Board exam.

13. Jack D. Walker, "The Goat Gland Surgeon: The Story of the Late John R. Brinkley," *Journal of the Kansas Medical Society* 57 (1956): pp. 749–55; Thomas Neville Bonner, *The Kansas Doctor: A Century of Pioneering* (Lawrence: University of Kansas Press, 1959), p. 80. At one point in the state's history, Kansas was considered "the plague spot of the nation in the indiscriminant licensing of doctors."

14. Lawrence Lowell, chairman, "The Final Report of the Commission on Med-

ical Education," Office of the Director of the Study, 1932: p. 3.

15. Shyrock, p. 60.

16. Ibid., pp. 62–4.

17. Editorial, *Journal of the American Medical Association* 89 (1927): p. 625.

18. William Allen Pusey, "The Disappearance of Doctors from Small Towns," *Journal of the American Medical Association* 88 (1927): p. 505.

19. Clement Wood, *The Life of a Man* (Kansas City: Goshen Publishing, 1934), pp. 93–100. Wood's biography was commissioned by Brinkley and contains numerous contradictions about the schools Brinkley attended prior to medical school. However, it is the main source about Brinkley's early life and the start of his career.

20. Ibid.

21. Theodore B. Schwartz, "Henry Harrower and the Turbulent Beginnings of Endocrinology," *Annals of Internal Medicine* 13 (1999): pp. 722; Lee, p. 31.

22. Lee, p. 31.

23. Ibid., p. 32; Carson, p. 34.

24. Wood, p. 93.

25. Lee, p. 32.

26. Helen Francis, "The Goat Gland Man," *Kansas Quarterly* 8 (1976): pp. 59–63. The movie commissioned by Brinkley was advertised in the *Los Angeles Record*, October 7, 1922. It was reported as telling the story of Billy Sittsworth.

27. Lee, p. 34.

28. Ibid. Mrs. Arfie Condray recalled, "Brinkley was a fine doctor and certainly was no quack as he was made out to be. He was a wonderful man." Arfie, age eighty-eight, was named Queen of the first Dr. Brinkley Day. *Junction City Union*, July 27, 1997, Geary County Historical Society, Junction City, Kansas. Brinkley file 2.

29. Wood, p. 115.

30. Carson, p. 37. Dr. Morris Fishbein, editor of the *Journal of the American Medical Association*, could not recall any article sent to the *Journal* by Brinkley.

31. John R. Brinkley, *The Brinkley Operation* (Chicago: Sydney B. Flower, 1922), p. 23.

32. Bureau of Investigation, "John R. Brinkley—Quack," *Journal of the American Medical Association* 90 (1928): p. 134. This article reveals several letterheads used by Brinkley over the past few years. In the letterhead labeled "Brinkley Research Laboratory," Minnie's name appears with an

M.D. degree; she was listed as an anesthetist. Surprisingly, it took Dr. Fishbein seven or eight years documenting Brinkley's practices, before he was labeled a "quack."

33. "Dr. Tobias Says: I'm Rejuvenated by Goat Glands," *Chicago Daily Tribune*, August 19, 1920.

34. Jean J. Du Bois (Tobias), *How to Win* (Chicago: Chicago Law School Press, 1929), pp. 242–4.

35. Death Notices, Jean J. Du Bois (John J. Tobias), *Chicago Daily Tribune*, July 12, 1932.

36. Wesley Staley, "Testimonial Letter," American Medical Association Archives 0099–07.

37. Brinkley, *The Brinkley Operation*, p. 12.

38. Rupert Billingham and Willys Silvers, *The Immunology of Transplantation* (Englewood Cliffs: Prentice Hall, 1971), p. 73.

39. Brinkley, *The Brinkley Operation*, p. 12.

40. John W. Gunn, Interview with Dr. Brinkley, "Life and Letters," Girard, Kansas, American Medical Association Archives 0096–04.

41. Sydney B. Flower, *The Goat Gland Operation Originated by Dr. J.R. Brinkley of Milford Kansas* (Chicago: New Thought Books, 1921), p. 82; Brinkley, *The Brinkley Operation*, p. 40. Brinkley boasted, "In the use of human glands Dr. Lydston is as supreme as I am in the use of goat glands."

42. Francis Chase, Jr., *The Sound and Fury: An Informal History of Broadcasting* (New York: Harper & Brothers, 1942), p. 61.

43. Edward Larusso, "The Goat Gland Film," *The Midnight Palace, midnight palace.com/article–goatgland.htm.*

44. Chase, p. 61; Lee, p. 62.

45. Lee, p. 74.

46. Walker, p. 752. Women were avid listeners to Brinkley's programs. This reference contains four letters from women with complaints.

47. Carson, p. 102.

48. Walter Davenport, "Gland Time in Kansas," *Colliers* (January 16, 1932): pp. 12–3.

49. Lee, p. 58. The advertisement for this rectal application of the emulsion stated that a satisfied user in Santa Ana, California, found this treatment resulted in improvement in the use of his right arm

and leg, presumably following a stroke. Of course, the passage of time may also have played a role in his recovery.

50. Chase, pp. 77–8.

51. Lee, p. 80; Carson, p. 103. The estimated income from just the pharmaceutical association came to between $10,000 and $14,000 per week.

52. W.A. Carr, M.D., interview with Ansel Harlan Resler, June 14, 1954, in "The Impact of John R. Brinkley on Broadcasting in the United States," PhD dissertation, Northwestern University, 1958, p. 24. Resler's dissertation is valuable because of the firsthand interviews he conducted with individuals who had worked for Brinkley or who had known him while he was still in Milford.

53. Wood, p. 218.

54. John R. Brinkley, *Shadows and Sunshine* (Milford, KS: J.R. Brinkley, 1923), pp. 22–63.

55. Ibid., p. 31.

56. Robert Morgan, "Borrow Life from a Goat? Transplanters Cause New Charlatanism to Flourish," *Dearborn Independent*, March 1, 1924.

57. Morris Fishbein, Editorial, "John R. Brinkley—Quack," *Journal of the American Medical Association* 90 (1928): pp. 134–7. It is surprising how many years it took Fishbein to label Brinkley as a quack.

58. Lee, pp. 92–3.

59. Carson, p. 103.

60. Lee, pp. 98–9.

61. Lee, p. 99; Chase, p. 72.

62. Lee, p. 103. The period from June 13, 1930, to February 21, 1931, allowed Brinkley to use his radio station for his political campaign.

63. Lee, 93–4.

64. Alexander B. Macdonald, cited in "Bureau of Investigation," *Journal of the American Medical Association* 94 (1930): pp. 1426–7.

65. Alexander B. Macdonald, *Kansas City Star*, July 16, 1930.

66. American Medical Association Archives 0097–02.

67. Ibid., 0096–06.

68. *Kansas City Star*, May 11, 1930; Lee, p. 88; R. Alton Lee, "Review of *Charlatan: America's Most Dangerous Huckster, the Man Who Pursued Him, and the Age of Flimflam*, by Pope Brock," *Kansas History* 31 (2008): p. 144.

69. Pope Brock, *Charlatan: America's Most Dangerous Huckster, the Man Who Pursued Him, and the Age of Flimflam* (New York: Crown Books, 2008), 154, 274.

70. Lee, p. 98. The opinion was delivered by Judge Rousseau A. Burch.

71. Carson, p. 149; Lee p. 111.

72. W.G. Clugston, *Rascals in Democracy* (New York: Richard R. Smith, 1941), p. 152.

73. Carson, p. 149.

74. Lee, p. 109.

75. Carson, pp. 150–1.

76. Kansas State History Library, Brinkley Collection 108–1–8. Two accounts of the surgery were provided by the press, one by W.G. Clugston from the *Kansas City Journal Post* and the other by Clif Stratton from the *Topeka Daily Capital*, both dated September 16, 1930. The accounts differ somewhat but are not contradictory. Stratton provided Mrs. Brinkley's remark.

77. Ibid.

78. Ibid. During the dissection of the vas deferens in one patient, Clugston heard Brinkley remark that the "vas got away from the pliers." What Brinkley probably meant by pliers was a tissue forceps, an instrument designed to hold tissue while the surgeon is dissecting it.

79. Carson, pp. 151–2.

80. Lee, p. 113.

81. Ibid., p. 116; Wood, pp. 260–1.

82. Lee, pp. 122–4.

83. *Fort Scott (Kansas) Daily-Monitor* June 6, 1930. American Medical Association Archives 0097–01.

84. Francis W. Schruben, "The Wizard of Milford," *Kansas History* 14 (1991): p. 238.

85. Lee, p. 122.

86. Ibid., p. 128.

87. Walker, p. 754; Lee, pp. 147–9.

88. Kansas State Board of Health—Division of Vital Statistics, Standard Certificate of Death, 31–2977, and 31–2978, American Medical Association Archives 0099–08.

89. Wood, p. 306.

90. Lee, p. 160.

91. Gene Fowler and Bill Crawford, *Border Radio: Quacks, Yodelers, Pitchmen, Psychics and Other Amazing Broadcasters of the American Airwaves* (Austin: University of Texas Press, 2002), p. 38; Lee, p. 161; Brock, p. 275.

92. Brinkley, *The Brinkley Operation*, pp. 30–1.

93. American Medical Association Archives, 0096–08.

94. Carson, pp. 203–4; "The Case of Brinkley vs. Fishbein," *Journal of the American Medical Association*, 112 (1939): p. 1960. Brinkley generated a gross income of about one million dollars in 1937; it was around eight hundred ten thousand dollars in 1938.

95. Current Comment, "Brinkley on the Brink," *Journal of the American Medical Association* 115 (1940): pp. 1368, 1655.

96. Morris Fishbein, "Modern Medical Charlatans," *Hygeia* 16 (February 1938): p. 172.

97. "The Case of Brinkley vs. Fishbein," *Journal of the American Medical Association* 112 (1939): pp. 1952–2288.

98. Ibid., p. 1952.

99. Ibid., pp. 1952–3; p. 2277–8; Lee, p. 230; John Thomas, "Diamond Studded John Richard Brinkley, The Goat Gland Broadcaster of Kansas," *Real America* (July 1933); American Medical Association Archives 0096–07.

100. Lee, p. 230.

101. Alexander B. Macdonald, *Kansas City Star*, June 15, 1930.

102. Resler, p. 235.

103. Ibid.

104. Macdonald, *Kansas City Star*, June 15, 1930.

105. John D'Amilio and Ester Freedman, *Intimate Matters: A History of Sexuality in America*, 2nd ed. (Chicago: University of Chicago Press, 1997), p. 233; Laura Davidov Hirshbein, "The Glandular Solution: Sex Masculinity, and Aging in the 1920s," *Journal of the History of Sexuality* 9 (2000): pp. 303–4.

106. Chase, p. 71.

107. John R. Brinkley, "Christmas Letter," December 24, 1932, Kansas State History Library, Brinkley collection 107–1-1. Mrs. Brinkley donated a number of items, including this letter, to the library.

108. Derrow Evans, "The Twilight of Minerva Brinkley," *Dallas Times Herald Magazine*, September 2, 1973.

109. David Kendall and Ralph Titus, "Goat Gland Doctor," Videocassette, Washburn University Library, Topeka, Kansas.

Chapter 8

1. William H. Helfand, *Quack, Quack, Quack: Nostrums in Ephemera & Books* (New York: Studley Press, 2002), pp. 13–4.

2. Roy Porter, *Health for Sale: Quackery in England 1660–1850* (Manchester: Manchester University Press, 1989), p. vii.

3. Ibid.

4. Ibid., p. vi.

5. James Harvey Young, *American Health Quackery* (Princeton: Princeton University Press, 1992), pp. 236–42.

6. American Medical Association Archives 0097–09.

7. Angus McLaren, *Impotence: A Cultural History* (Chicago: University of Chicago Press, 2007), pp. 135–7. Several dietary sources are listed for rejuvenating "exhausted men over forty." These include "milk, hot chocolate for breakfast, steak for lunch, bloody roast beef for dinner accompanied by rocket, artichokes, and bottles of burgundy." Dietary recommendations were also described by Martin Gardner, *Fads and Fallacies in the Name of Science* (New York: Dover, 1957), p. 244. These include eggs and foods which resemble genital organs such as "asparagus, celery, onions, and oysters."

8. Young, *American Health Quackery*, p. 237.

9. Gardner, p. 186.

10. Young, *American Health Quackery*, p. 38, 240. The notorious quack Albert Abrams was able to convince the writer Upton Sinclair and the actor Charlie Chaplin that a perfectly worthless device could diagnose variety of diseases. Sinclair then praised Abrams for his "most revolutionary discovery of this or any other age."

11. Young, *American Health Quackery*, pp. 236–42.

12. Ibid.

13. Young, *American Health Quackery*, p. 241.

14. James Harvey Young, *The Medical Messiahs* (Princeton: Princeton University Press, 1967), pp. 26–7.

15. Brinkley, *The Brinkley Operation*, pp. 23–4.

16. Thomas T. Perls, "Anti-Aging Quackery: Human Growth Hormone and Tricks of the Trade—More Dangerous than Ever," *Journal of Gerontology: Biological Sciences* 59A (2004): pp. 682–91.

17. Ibid., p. 683.

18. Young, *American Health Quackery*, p. 237.

19. Arthur Cramp, *Nostrums and Quackery*, vol. 2 (Chicago: American Medical Association, 1921), pp. 721–3.

20. Young, *The Medical Messiahs*, pp. 66–7. Young emphasized that the Post

Office Department was the first government agency to combat medical quackery, by halting use of the mail by quacks.

21. The Propaganda for Reform, "P. Presto Company, the Government Stops Oregon Fraud," *Journal of the American Medical Association* 73 (1919): p. 1302.

22. Ibid.

23. Morris Fishbein, *Fads and Quackery in Healing* (New York: Blue Ribbon Books, 1932), pp. 236–8.

24. Ibid.

25. Ibid.

26. *University of California, Berkeley Wellness Letter*, February 7, 2015. The cost of these health products is estimated at $28 billion dollars a year.

27. Robert L. Park, *Voodoo Science: The Road from Foolishness to Fraud* (New York: Oxford University Press, 2000), pp. 48–9; Perls, p. 682.

28. Park, pp. 48–9.

Chapter 9

1. Mark Twain, *A Connecticut Yankee in King Arthur's Court* (New York: Charles L. Webster & Company, 1889), p. 337. Twain used the above phrase to explain a site where a girl herding geese was said to have witnessed the Virgin Mary. A chapel was built there containing a painting depicting this visionary occurrence. Subsequently, thousands of those who were lame and sick came to pray before the chapel and were cured. "I saw cripples whom I had seen around Camelot for years on crutches, arrive and pray before the picture, put down their crutches and walk off without a limp," was how the Connecticut Yankee described the scene.

2. Andrea J. Cussons, Chotoo Bhgat, Stephen J. Fletcher, and John P. Walsh, "Brown-Séquard Revisited: A Lesson from History on the Placebo Effect of Androgen Treatment," *Medical Journal of Australia* 177 (2002): pp. 678–9.

3. Charles Édouard Brown-Séquard, "The Effects on Man by Subcutaneous Injections of a Liquid Obtained from Testicles of Animals," *Lancet* (July 20, 1889): pp. 105–7.

4. Steven W.J. Lamberts, "Endocrinology and Aging," in *Williams Textbook of Endocrinology*, eds. Shlomo Melmed, Kenneth S. Polansky, P. Reed Larsen, and Henry M. Kronenberg (Philadelphia: Saunders Elsevier, 2011), pp. 1219–33. This chapter describes the decline of testosterone in aging men and its treatment.

5. Louis Lasagna, "The Placebo Effect," *Journal of Clinical Immunology* 78 (1986): pp. 162–5; Anne Harrington, *The Cure Within: A History of Mind-Body Medicine* (New York: W.W. Norton, 2008), 62–3.

6. Lasagna, p. 161.

7. Arthur K. Shapiro and Elaine Shapiro, "The Placebo: Is It Much Ado About Nothing?" in *The Placebo Effect*, ed. Anne Harrington (Cambridge: Harvard University Press, 1999), pp. 12–3.

8. Ted Kaptchuk, "Powerful Placebo: The Dark Side of the Randomized Controlled Trial," *Lancet* 351 (1998): pp. 1722–5; Donald D. Price and Howard L. Fields, "The Contribution of Desire and Expectation in Placebo Anesthesia: Implications for New Research Strategies," in *The Placebo Effect*, ed. Anne Harrington, pp. 117–31; Fabrizio Benedetti, *The Placebo Effects: Understanding the Mechanisms in Health and Disease* (New York: Oxford University Press, 2000), pp. 38–9; Daniel Moerman, "Meaningful Placebos—Controlling the Uncontrollable," *New England Journal of Medicine* 365 (July 14, 2011): pp. 171–2.

9. Kaptchuk, p. 1722.

10. Conference on Therapy, "The Use of Placebos in Therapy," *New York State Medical Journal* 46 (1946): pp. 1718–27.

11. Ibid., p. 1719.

12. George Bernard Shaw, *The Doctor's Dilemma* (New York: Dodd, Mead, 1941), pp. 20–1.

13. Alan G. Johnson, "Surgery as a Placebo," *Lancet* 344 (1994): pp. 1140–2.

14. Moerman, pp. 171–2.

15. Rita F. Redberg, "Sham Controls in Medical Devices," *New England Journal of Medicine* 371 (2014): pp. 892–3.

16. Ibid.

17. Gunver S. Keinle and Helmut Keinle, "The Powerful Placebo Effect: Fact of Fiction?" *Journal of Clinical Epidemiology* 50 (1997): pp. 1311–8.

18. Henry K. Beecher, "The Powerful Placebo," *Journal of the American Medical Association* 159 (1955): pp. 1602–6.

19. Howard A. Fink, R. Macdonald, I.R. Rutkus, D.B. Nelson, and T.J. Wilt, "Sildenafil for Male Erectile Dysfunction: A Systemic Review and Metanalysis," *Archives of Internal Medicine* 162 (2002): pp. 1349–60; Meika Loe, *The Rise of Viagra* (New York: New York University Press, 2004), p.

54. The author concluded that "just the idea of Viagra (sildenafil) may be effective in some patients."

20. H. Padma Nathan, "Treatment of Men with Erectile Dysfunction with Transurethal Alprostadil," *New England Journal of Medicine* 336 (1997): pp. 1–7.

21. Androgel Prescribing Information, "Designed with a Man in Mind," AbbVie Inc., North Chicago, IL, 60064.

22. Richard Kradin, *The Placebo Response and the Power of Unconscious Healing* (New York: Routledge, 2008), pp. 83–5.

23. Fabrizio Benedetti, "Mental and Behavioral Disorders," chapter 5 in *Placebo Effects: Understanding the Mechanisms in Health and Disease* (New York: Oxford University Press, 2009 (see illustrations).

24. Ibid., chapter 5.

25. "Tell of Gains Made in Fight on Old Age," *New York Times*, August 24, 1929.

26. Kradin, pp. 134–5.

27. Serge Voronoff, *Rejuvenation by Grafting*, pp. 21–3.

28. Nicholas L. Tilney, *Transplant: From Myth to Reality* (New Haven: Yale University Press, 2003), pp. 33–4. In this relatively brief account of the gland grafting experience, the author does not include the continuation of Dr. Brinkley's rejuvenation practice, using vasectomy instead of goat testicles. Brinkley continued to acquire considerable income helped by his advertising over his radio station in Mexico.

29. Ted J. Kaptchuk and Franklin G. Miller, "Placebo Effects in Medicine," *New England Journal of Medicine* 373 (July 2, 2015): pp. 8–9. This article offers an excellent summary of current research on placebos.

30. Josephine P. Briggs and Jack Killen, "Perspectives on Complementary and Alternative Medicine Research," *Journal of the American Medical Association* 310 (2013): pp. 691–2.

Chapter 10

1. George W. Corner, "The Early History of Oestrogenic Hormones," *The Journal of Endocrinology* 31 (1965): p. iii.

2. Ibid., p. v.

3. Ibid., p. vii.

4. Ibid.

5. Hans H. Simmer, "Robert Tuttle Morris (1857–1945): A Pioneer in Ovarian Transplants," *Obstetrics and Gynecology* 35 (1970): pp. 314–27.

6. Ibid., p. 315.

7. Ibid., pp. 319–20.

8. Ibid., pp. 318–9.

9. Robert T. Morris, "A Case of Heteroplastic Ovarian Grafting Followed by a Pregnancy and Delivery of a Living Child," *Medical Record* 69 (1906): p. 697; Simmer, pp. 319–20.

10. Simmer, p. 320.

11. Ibid., p. 322.

12. Franklin H. Martin, "Ovarian Transplantation," *Surgery, Gynecology & Obstetrics* 35 (1922): pp. 573–85.

13. Corner, p. v.

14. Ibid., p. vi.

15. Ibid., p. ix.

16. Ibid.

17. Ibid., p. x.

18. Ibid., p. xi; Elizabeth Siegel Watkins, *The Estrogen Elixir* (Baltimore: Johns Hopkins University Press, 2007), pp. 11–2.

19. Edgar Allen and Edward A. Doisy, "The Extraction and Some Properties of an Ovarian Hormone," *Journal of Biological Chemistry* 61 (1924): pp. 711–27.

20. Watkins, p. 12.

21. Adolf Butenandt, Nobel Lectures, Chemistry 1922–41 (Amsterdam: Elsevier, 1966): Nobel Prize.org.

22. Watkins, p. 47.

23. Ibid., pp. 32–4.

24. Ibid., pp. 48–50.

25. Ibid., p. 49.

26. Ibid., pp. 93–4.

27. Ibid., pp. 28, 216.

28. Ibid., pp. 209–11.

29. Ibid.

30. Marcelle I. Cedars and Michele Evans, "Menopause," in *Danforth's Obstetrics and Gynecology*, 10th ed., edited by Ronald S. Gibbs, Beth Y. Karlan, Arthur F. Haney, and Ingrid Nygaard (Philadelphia: Lippincott, Williams & Wilkins, 2008), pp. 725–41.

31. Ibid., p. 730.

32. Ibid. p. 732.

33. Ibid., pp. 736–7.

34. Ibid.

35. Ibid.

36. Ibid., pp. 738–9.

37. Howard N. Hodis, Wendy J. Mack, Victor W. Henderson, et al., "Vascular Effects of Early versus Late Postmenopausal Treatment with Estradiol," *New England Journal of Medicine* 374 (2016): pp. 1221–31; John F. Kearney and Caren G. Solomon,

"Postmenopausal Hormone Therapy and Atherosclerosis—Time Is of the Essence," *New England Journal of Medicine* 374 (2016): pp. 1279–80.

38. F. Cory Cunningham, Kenneth J. Levene, Steven L. Bloom, John C. Hauth, Dwight J. Rouse and Catherine Y. Spong, "Contraception," in *Williams Obstetrics*, 23rd ed. (New York: McGraw Hill Medical, 2010), pp. 673–4.

39. Carl Djerassi, *This Man's Pill* (Oxford University Press, 2001), pp. 16–9; Obituary, "Carl Djerassi, 91, a Creator of the Birth Control Pill, Dies," *New York Times*, February 1, 2015. The obituary provides a brief summary of Djerassi's long, distinguished scientific career.

40. A.W. Makepeace, George L. Weinstein and Maurice H. Friedman, "The Effect of Progesterin and Progesterone on Ovulation in the Rabbit," *Proceedings of the Society for Experimental Biology and Medicine* 35 (1936): pp. 269–70.

41. Jonathan Eig, *The Birth of the Pill* (New York: W.W. Norton, 2014), pp. 21–3.

42. Ibid., p. 3.

43. Ibid., pp. 30–1.

44. Ibid., p. 33.

45. Ibid., pp. 90–1; Elaine Tyler May, *America and the Pill* (New York: Basic Books, 2010), p. 21.

46. Eig, p. 94.

47. Ibid., p. 103.

48. Ibid., pp. 104–5.

49. Djerassi, pp. 50–1.

50. Ibid.

51. Eig, pp. 138–9.

52. Ibid., p. 258.

53. Ibid., p. 159.

54. Ibid., p. 242.

55. May, pp. 23–4.

56. Eig, pp. 291–2.

57. May, p. 34.

58. Ibid., p. 144.

59. Ibid., p. 168, 321.

60. Eig, p. 5.

61. May, p. 168.

Chapter 11

1. T.F. Gallagher and Fred C. Koch, "The Testicular Hormone," *Journal of Biological Chemistry* 84 (1929): pp. 495–500.

2. Eberhard Nieschlag, "History of Testosterone," Endocrine Abstracts.org (2005) 10 S2.

3. Nobelprize.org, "Nobel Lectures, Chemistry, 1922–41" (Amsterdam: Elsevier, 1966).

4. John Hoberman, *Testosterone Dreams* (Berkeley: University of California Press, 2005), pp. 55–7.

5. Charles W. Lloyd and Joan Fredericks, "Testosterone Cyclopentylpropionate: Long Acting Androgen," *Journal of Clinical Endocrinology* 11 (1951): pp. 724–7.

6. Walter R. Stokes, "Sexual Function in the Aging Male," *Geriatrics* 6 (1951): p. 304–8.

7. Maurice A. Lesser, Samuel N. Vose and Grant M. Dixey, "Effect of Testosterone Propionate on Prostate Gland of Patients over 45," *Journal of Clinical Endocrinology* 16 (1955): pp. 297–300.

8. J.S. Tenover, "Effects of Testosterone Supplementation in the Aging Male," *Journal of Clinical Endocrinology* 75 (1992): pp. 1092–8.

9. Rabih. A. Hijazi and Glenn R. Cunningham, "Andropause: Is Androgen Replacement Therapy Indicated for the Aging Male?" *Annual Review of Medicine* 56 (2005): pp. 117–132.

10. Ibid., p. 122.

11. Ibid., p. 121–2.

12. Andrea M. Isidori and Andrea Lenzi, "Testosterone Replacement Therapy: What We Know is Not Enough," *Mayo Clinic Proceedings* 82 (2007): pp. 11–13.

13. Enrique R. Bolona, Andrea D. Coviello, Thomas G. Travison, et al., "Testosterone Use in Men with Sexual Dysfunction: A Systemic Review and Meta-analysis of Randomized Placebo-controlled Trials," *Mayo Clinic Proceedings* 82 (2007): pp. 21–8.

14. Sergio A. Moreno and Abraham Morgentaler, "Hormonal Evaluation and Therapy in Erectile Dysfunction," in *Contemporary Treatment of Erectile Dysfunction*, ed. Kevin McVary (New York: Humana Press/Springer Science + Business Media, 2011), pp. 161–73.

15. Shehzad Basafia, Andrea D. Coviello, Thomas G. Tavison, et al., "Adverse Events Associated with Testosterone Administration," *New England Journal of Medicine* 363 (2010): pp. 109–22.

16. William J. Bremner, "Testosterone Deficiency and Replacement in Older Men," *New England Journal of Medicine* 363 (2010): p. 189–91.

17. Frederick C.W. Wu, Abdelouahid Tajar, Jennifer M. Beynon, et al., "Identification of Late-Onset Hypogonadism in

Middle-Aged and Elderly Men," *New England Journal of Medicine* 363 (2010): pp. 123–135.

18. Ibid., pp. 133–4.

19. Joel S. Finkelstein, Hang Lee, Sherri-Ann Burnett-Brown, et al., "Gonadal Steroids and Body Composition, Strength, and Sexual function in Men," *New England Journal of Medicine* 369 (2013): p. 1011–22.

20. Ibid., p. 1018.

21. Ibid., pp. 1018–9.

22. Tobias S. Kohler, "Testosterone," *AUA* (American Urological Association) *News* 19 (2014): pp. 1, 6–7.

23. Rudy M. Haddad, Cassie C. Kennedy, Sean M. Caples, et al., "Testosterone and Cardiovascular Risk in Men: A Systemic Review and Meta-Analysis of Randomized, Placebo-Controlled Trials," *Mayo Clinic Proceedings* 82 (2007): pp. 29–39.

24. Alvaro Morales, "Androgen Deficiency in the Aging Male," chapter 29 in *Campbell-Walsh Urology*, 10th ed., eds. Alan J. Wein, Louis R. Kovousi, Andrew C. Novak, Alan W. Partin, and Craig A. Peters (Philadelphia: Elsevier-Saunders, 2012), p. 819.

25. Kohler, p. 7.

26. Cynthia M. Kuhn, "Anabolic Steroids," *Recent Progress in Hormone Research* 57 (2002): pp. 411–29.

27. Jean D. Wilson, "Androgen Abuse by Athletes," *Endocrine Review* 9 (1988): pp. 181–91; John M. Hoberman and Charles E. Yesalis, "The History of Synthetic Testosterone," *Scientific American* (February 1995): pp. 77–81.

28. Ibid.

29. Brian Costa and Andrew Grossman, "Baseball Steroid Supplier is Charged," *Wall Street Journal*, August 6, 2014, A3.

30. Kuhn, 428.

31. David Von Drehle, "Feeling Deflated? The 'Low-T' Industry Wants to Pump You Up," *Time*, August 15, 2014, pp. 37–43; David D. Federman and Geoffrey A. Walford, "Is Male Menopause Real?" *Newsweek*, January 15, 2007, pp. 58–60.

32. Martin Miner, "Mispreconceptions and Myths of Testosterone Abuse in Middle Age," *AUA News* (September 2014): pp. 14, 20.

33. Ibid., p. 20.

34. Ajay K. Nangia, "Testosterone Is Being Abused in Middle Age," *AUA News* (September 2014): pp. 14–5, 20.

35. Ibid., p. 20.

36. Editorial, "Testosterone-Replacement Therapy," *New England Journal of Medicine* 371 (2014): p. 2032; Ronald Swerdloff, "Recommend Testosterone-Replacement Therapy," *New England Journal of Medicine* 371 (2014): p. 2033; Bradley D. Anawalt, "Recommend Against Testosterone-Replacement Therapy," *New England Journal of Medicine* 371 (2014): pp. 2033–4.

37. Mark B. Garnick, "Testosterone Replacement Therapy Faces FDA Scrutiny," *Journal of the American Medical Association* 313, (2015): p. 563–4.

38. Peter J. Snyder, Shalender Bhasin, Glenn R. Cunningham, et al., "Effects of Testosterone Treatment in Elderly Men," *New England Journal of Medicine* 374 (2016): pp. 611–23.

39. Eric S. Orwoll, "Establishing a Framework—Does Testosterone Supplementation Help Older Men?" *New England Journal of Medicine* 374 (2016): p. 682–3.

Chapter 12

1. Adam Leith Gollner, *The Book of Immortality* (New York: Scribner, 2013), p. 124; Sam Anderson, "Hope Springs Eternal," *New York Times Health Issue*, October 26, 2014, pp. 32–5.

2. Gollner, p. 104.

3. Ibid., p. 106.

4. Ibid., pp. 114–5.

5. Gunnar Heydenreich, *Lucas Cranach the Elder* (Amsterdam: Amsterdam University Press, 2007), p. 180; Alexander Stepanov, *Lucas Cranach the Elder* (Bournemouth, England: Parkstone Press, 1997), p. 67. The image was obtained from the Art Renewal Center, Port Reading, New Jersey. The original resides in the Staatliche Museen, Berlin-Dalem, Germany.

6. Gollner, p. 123.

7. Ponce de Leon, Wikipedia.org.

8. Gollner, p. 143.

9. Ibid.

10. Anderson, p. 34.

11. Ibid.

12. Ibid., pp. 34–5; Ocalaflorida.com.

13. Anderson, p. 35.

14. Gollner, 125–8.

15. St. Augustinerecord.com/stories.

16. Gollner, pp. 127–8.

17. Fountainofyouthflorida.com; Gollner, p. 134.

18. Gollner, pp. 138–9.
19. Ibid., p. 139.

Chapter 13

1. Ansel Harlan Resler, "The Impact of John R. Brinkley on Broadcasting in the United States." PhD diss., Northwestern University, 1958, p. 180.
2. Resler, p. 219.
3. R. Alton Lee, *The Bizarre Careers of John R. Brinkley* (Lexington: University Press of Kentucky, 2002), p. 46.
4. Ibid.
5. Alexander B. Macdonald, *Kansas City Star*, June 15, 1930.
6. Lee, pp. 83–4.
7. Letter from the American Consul, Piedras Negras, Mexico, to Secretary of State, November 20, 1933. State Department Files, cited in Resler, p. 249.
8. Interview with W.A. Carr, M.D., Junction City, Kansas, June 16, 1954, cited in Resler, p. 249.
9. Resler, p. 257.
10. Roy Porter, *Bodies Politic: Disease, Death, and Doctors in Britain, 1650–1900* (London: Reaktion Books, 2001), p. 22; Elizabeth Lane Furdell, *Publishing and Medicine in Early Modern England* (Rochester: University of Rochester Press, 2002), p. 4–11.
11. Furdell, pp. 23, 43.
12. Ibid., 49.
13. Andrew Wear, *Knowledge and Practice in English Medicine, 1550–1680* (Cambridge: Cambridge University Press, 2000), pp. 40–2. Wear cites that there were 238 medical books published in the mid-17th century, thirty-one of which were in Latin.
14. Wear, p. 46
15. Furdell, p. 146.
16. Ibid., p. 137.
17. Wear, pp. 46, 68–9.
18. Ibid., pp. 434–6; Porter, pp. 201–3.
19. Claire Hoertz Badaracco, *Prescribing Faith: Medicine, Media, and Religion in American Culture* (Waco, TX: Baylor University Press, 2007), p. 27.
20. Richard Weinmeyer, "Direct-to-Consumer Advertising of Drugs," *AMA Journal of Ethics 15* (November 2013): pp. 954–9.
21. Ibid.
22. Janet Heinrich, United States General Accounting Office: Report to Congressional Requesters, Prescription Drugs (October 2002), pp. 1–3; U.S. Food and Drug Administration: Prescription Drug Advertising [accessed 11/02/2015]; www. gov?Drugs?ResourcesForYou/Consumers/Prescription Drug Advertising.
23. Trevor A. Fisk, *Advertising Health Services: What Works—What Fails.* (Chicago: Pluribus Press, 1986), pp. 72, 127.
24. Ibid., p. 81.
25. Random Facts: Interesting Facts about Advertising, #38; http://facts.random history.com/interesting-facts-about-advertising.html [accessed 11/14/2015].
26. Fisk, p. 170.
27. Ibid., pp. 199–200.
28. Jon C. Schommer and Lewis H. Glinert, *A Screenful of Sugar?* (New York: Peter Lang, 2014), p. 86.
29. U.S. Food and Drug Administration, Basics of Drug Ads [accessed 1/6/2016]. http://www.fda.gov/Drugs/ResourcesFor You/Consumers/PrescriptionDrug/ Advertising/ucm072077.htm.
30. U.S. Food and Drug Administration, Keeping Watch Over Direct-to-Consumer Ads (May 10, 2010), http://www.fda.gov/ ForConsumers/ConsumerUpdates/ucm 107170.htm.
31. U.S. Food and Drug Administration, Prescription Drug Advertising: Questions to Ask Yourself [accessed 1/6/2016]. http:// www.fda.gov/Drugs/ResourcesForYou/ Consumers/PrescriptionDrugAdvertising/ ucm1915.htm.
32. Julie M. Donohue, Marisa Cervasco, and Meredith B. Rosenthal, "A Decade of Direct-to-Consumer Advertising," *New England Journal of Medicine* 357 (2007): p. 673–81.
33. U.S. Food and Drug Administration, The Impact of Direct-to-Consumer Advertising (2004). http://www.fda.gov/Drugs/ ResourcesForYou/Consumers/ucm143562. htm.
34. Badaracco, 160.
35. United States General Accounting Office Report to Congressional Requesters, p. 14.
36. Marcia Angell, *The Truth About the Drug Companies* (New York: Random House, 2004), xii.
37. Marcia Angell, "Relationships of the Drug Industry: Keep at Arm's Length," *British Medical Journal* 338 (2009): p. 222.
38. Schommer and Glinert, p. 5.
39. Ibid., p. 1.
40. Ray Moynihan and Alan Cassels, *Selling Sickness: How the World's Biggest*

Pharmaceutical Companies are Turning Us All into Patients (New York: Nation Books, 2005), p. x.

41. Schommer and Glinert, p. 16.

42. Ibid.

43. Moynihan and Cassels, xvii.

44. Ibid., p. 4, 87.

45. http://www.heart.org/HEARTORG/Conditions/More/CardiacRehab/Taking-Care-Of-Yourself/UCM307 (1–13-2015); http://www.ama-assn.org/ama/pub/news/2015–11-09-prioritize-blood-pressure-control.page.

46. Ibid.

47. Carl Elliot, *Better Than Well* (New York: W.W. Norton, 2003), pp. 230–1; Moynihan and Cassels, pp. 124–5.

48. Elliot, pp. 230–1; Moynihan and Cassels, p. 64.

49. Elliot, pp. 54, 75; Moynihan and Cassels, p. 64.

50. Moynihan and Cassels, p. 164.

51. Ibid., p. 99.

52. Elliot, p. xvi.

53. Ibid., p. 52.

54. Ibid., p. 54.

55. Ibid., p. 75.

56. Ibid., p. 75.

57. Ibid., p. 123.

58. Elizabeth D. Kantor, Colin D. Rehm, Jennifer S. Haas, et al., "Trends in Prescription Drug Use Among Adults in the United States from 1999–2012," *Journal of the American Medical Association* 314 (2015): pp. 1818–31.

59. Ibid., p. 1825.

60. John Russell, "AMA Calls for Ban on Ads that Pitch Drugs, Devices," *Chicago Tribune,* November 18, 2015.

61. Elizabeth Rosenthal, "Cure," *New York Times, Sunday Review,* February 28, 2016.

62. Russell, *Chicago Tribune.*

63. Peter Loftus, "Ads for Costly Drugs Get Airtime," *Wall Street Journal*, February 17, 2016, B1.

64. Russell.

65. Loftus.

66. Russell.

67. Peter B. Bach, "New Math on Drug Cost-Effectiveness," *New England Journal of Medicine* 373 (November 5, 2015): pp. 1797–8.

68. Susanna Every-Palmer, Rishi Duggal, and David B. Menkes, "Direct-to-Consumer Advertising of Prescription Medicine in New Zealand," *New Zealand Medical Journal* 127 (2014): pp. 102–110.

69. Jacqueline M. Barber and Kevin P. Sheehy, "Uptake of New Medicines in New Zealand," *New Zealand Medical Journal* 128 (2015): pp. 10–20.

70. Every-Palmer.

71. Ibid.

72. Barber, pp. 10–1.

73. Ibid., pp. 17–8.

74. Ibid.

75. Ibid.

76. Ibid., p. 16.

Bibliography

Books

Abrams, Roger E. *The Dark Side of the Diamond.* Boston: Rounder Books, 2007.

Allen, Fredrick Lewis. *Only Yesterday: An Informal History of the 1920s.* New York: Harper & Brothers, 1931.

Ameringer, Carl F. *State Medical Boards and the Politics of Public Protection.* Baltimore: Johns Hopkins University Press, 1999.

Aminoff, Michael J. *Brown-Séquard: A Visionary of Science.* New York: Raven Press, 1993.

Benedetti, Fabrizio. *Placebo Effects: Understanding the Mechanisms in Health and Disease.* New York: Oxford University Press, 2009.

Billingham, Rupert, and Willys Silvers. *The Immunology of Transplantation.* Englewood Cliffs, NJ: Prentice Hall, 1971.

Bliss, Michael. *The Discovery of Insulin, 25th ed.* Chicago: University of Chicago Press, 2007.

_____. *William Osler: A Life in Medicine.* New York: Oxford University Press, 1999.

Bonner, Neville. *The Kansas Doctor: A Century of Pioneering.* Lawrence: University of Kansas Press, 1959.

Carson, Gerald. *The Roguish World of Doctor Brinkley.* New York: Holt, Rinehart & Winston, 1960.

Casey, Robert J. *More Interesting People.* New York: Bobbs-Merrell, 1947.

Cedars, Marcelle, and Michele Evans. "Menopause." In *Danforth's Obstetrics and Gynecology*, 10th ed. Philadelphia: Lippincott Williams & Wilkins, 2008.

Chase, Francis Jr. *The Sound and Fury: An Informal History of Broadcasting.* New York: Harper & Brothers, 1942.

Clugston, W.G. *Rascals in Democracy.* New York: Richard R. Smith, 1941.

Cole, Thomas R. *The Journey of Life: A Cultural History of Aging in America.* New York: Cambridge University Press, 1992.

Corners, George. *Rejuvenation: How Steinach Makes People Young Again.* New York: Seltzer, 1923.

Cramp, Arthur. *Nostrums and Quackery*, vols. 1, 2. Chicago: American Medical Association, 1921.

Bibliography

Cunningham, F. Cary, Kenneth J. Leveno, Steven L. Bloom, et al. "Contraception." In *Williams Obstetrics*, 23rd ed. New York: McGraw-Hill Medical, 2010.

Cushing, Harvey. *The Life of Sir William Osler*, vols.1, 2. Oxford: Clarendon Press, 1925.

Davis, Loyal. *Neurological Surgery*. Philadelphia: Lea & Febiger, 1936.

Dedmon, Emmett. *Fabulous Chicago*. New York: Random House, 1953.

D'Eilio, John D., and Estell Freedman. *Intimate Matters: A History of Sexuality in America*. Chicago: University of Chicago Press, 1997.

Djurassi, Carl. *This Man's Pill*. Oxford: Oxford University Press, 2014.

DuBois, John J. *How to Win*. Chicago: Chicago Law School Press, 1929.

Eig, Jonathan. *Birth of the Pill*. New York: W.W. Norton, 2014.

Feldman, Martha. *The Castrato*. Oakland: University of California Press, 2015.

Fishbein, Morris. *An Autobiography*. Garden City: Doubleday, 1969.

_____. *Fads and Quackery in Healing*. New York: Blue Ribbon Books, 1937.

Flower, Sydney B. *The Goat Gland Operation Originated by Dr. J.R. Brinkley of Milford Kansas*. Chicago: New Thought Books, 1921.

Forth, Christopher. *Masculinity in the Modern West*. New York: Palgrave Macmillan, 2007.

Foster, Robert Fitzroy. *W.B. Yeats: A Life, the Arch Poet 1915–1939*. Oxford: Oxford University Press, 2003.

Friedlander, Max J., and Jacob Rosenberg. *The Paintings of Lucas Cranach*. New York: Cornell University Press, 1978.

Fulton, John F. *Selected Readings in the History of Physiology*, 2nd ed. Springfield: Charles C. Thomas, 1966.

Gardner, Martin. *Fads and Fallacies in the Name of Science*. New York: Dover, 1957.

Gollner, Adam Leith. *The Book of Immortality*. New York: Scribner, 2013.

Graebner, William. *A History of Retirement*. New Haven: Yale University Press, 1980.

Hamilton, David. *The Monkey Gland Affair*. London: Catto & Windus, 1980.

Haycock, David Boyd. *Mortal Coil: A Short History of Living Longer*. New Haven: Yale University Press, 2008.

Helfand, William H. *Quack, Quack, Quack: Nostrums in Ephemera and Books*. New York: Studley Press, 2002.

Hill, John. *The Old Man's Guide to Health and Longer Life with Rules for Diet, Exercise, and Physic*, 5th ed. London: R. Baldwin and J. Ridley, 1764.

Hoberman, John. *Testosterone Dreams*. Berkeley: University of California Press, 2005.

Kradin, Richard. *The Placebo Response and the Power of Unconscious Healing*. New York: Routledge, 2008.

Lederer, Susan E. *Flesh and Blood: Transplantation and Blood Transfusion in Twentieth Century America*. New York: Oxford University Press, 2008.

Lee, R. Alton. *The Bizarre Careers of John R. Brinkley*. Lexington: University of Kentucky Press, 2002.

Leider, Emily Wortis. *California's Daughter: Gertrude Atherton and Her Times*. Stanford: Stanford University Press, 1991.

Loe, Meika. *The Rise of Viagra*. New York: New York University Press, 2004.

Bibliography

Lydston, G. Frank. *Impotence and Sterility with Aberrations of the Sexual Function and Sex Gland Implantation.* Chicago: Riverton Press, 1917.
_____. *Surgical Diseases of the Genitourinary Tract.* Philadelphia: F.A. Davis, 1889.
McGrady, Patrick. *The Youth Doctors.* New York: Coward-McCann, 1968.
McLaren, Angus. *Impotence: A Cultural History.* Chicago: University of Chicago Press, 2005.
McVary, Kevin, ed. *Contemporary Treatment of Erectile Dysfunction.* New York: Humana Press/Springer Science + Business Media, 2011.
Olmsted, J.M.D. *Charles Edward Brown-Séquard: A Nineteenth Century Neurologist and Endocrinologist.* Baltimore: Johns Hopkins University Press, 1946.
Osler, William. *Aequanimitas.* Philadelphia: Blakiston, 1947.
Park, Robert L. *Voodoo Science: The Road from Foolishness to Fraud.* New York: Oxford University Press, 2000.
Porter, Roy. *Health for Sale: Quackery in England 1660–1850.* Manchester: Manchester University Press, 1989.
Price, Catherine. *Vitamania.* New York: Penguin Press, 2015.
Resler, Ansel Harlan. "The Impact of John R. Brinkley on Broadcasting in the United States." PhD dissertation, Northwestern University, 1958.
Romm, Sharon. *The Unwelcome Intruder: Freud's Struggle with Cancer.* New York: Praeger, 1983.
Sayers, Dorothy. *The Unpleasantness at the Bellona Club.* London: Victor Gollancz, 1972.
Schlich, Thomas. *The Origins of Organ Transplantation.* Rochester: University of Rochester Press, 2010.
Schuster, David C. *Neurasthenic Nation.* New Brunswick: Rutgers University Press, 2011.
Shyrock, Richard Harrison. *Medical Licensing in America, 1650–1965.* Baltimore: Johns Hopkins University Press, 1967.
Solberg, Winton U. *Reforming Medical Education.* Urbana: University of Illinois Press, 2009.
Stanley, Leo L. *Men at their Worst.* New York: Appleton-Century, 1940.
_____. *My Most Unforgettable Convicts.* Winnipeg: Greywood Publishing, 1967.
Steinach, Eugen. *Sex and Life.* New York: Viking, 1940.
Thorek, Max. *The Human Testis.* Philadelphia: J.B. Lippincott, 1924.
_____. *A Surgeon's World.* Philadelphia: Lippincott, 1943.
Tilney, Nicholas L. *Transplant: From Myth to Reality.* New Haven: Yale University Press, 2003.
Twain, Mark (Samuel Clemens). *A Connecticut Yankee in King Arthur's Court.* New York: Charles L. Webster Company, 1889.
Vice Commission of Chicago. *Social Evil in Chicago.* Chicago: Gunthorp-Warren, 1911.
Voronoff, Serge. *Life: A Study of the Means of Restoring Vital Energy and Prolonging Life.* New York: E.P. Dutton, 1920.
_____. *Rejuvenation by Grafting.* London: George Allen & Unwin, 1925.
Watkins, Elizabeth Siegel. *The Estrogen Elixir.* Baltimore: Johns Hopkins University Press, 2007.
Wood, Clement. *Life of a Man.* Kansas City: Goshorn Press, 1934.

Bibliography

Young, James Harvey. *American Health Quackery*. Princeton: Princeton University Press, 1992.
_____. *The Medical Messiahs*. Princeton: Princeton University Press, 1967.

Journals

Acta historica scientiarm naturalium et medicination
American Journal of Physiology
American Medicine
Annals of Internal Medicine
Annual Review of Medicine
Archives of Internal Medicine
Boston Medical and Surgical Journal
British Journal of Surgery
British Medical Journal
Bulletin of the History of Medicine
California State Journal of Medicine
Endocrinology
Geriatrics
Gerontology
Hygeia
Illinois State Medical Journal
International Clinics
Kansas Quarterly
Journal of Biological Chemistry
Journal of Clinical Endocrinology
Journal of Clinical Endocrinology and Metabolism
Journal of Clinical Epidemiology
Journal of Endocrinology
Journal of the Australian Medical Association
Journal of the History of Medicine and Allied Sciences
Journal of the History of Sexuality
Journal of the Kansas Medical Society
Journal of Urology
Lancet
Mayo Clinic Proceedings
Medical Journal of Australia
Nature
New England Journal of Medicine
New York Medical Journal
New York State Journal of Medicine
Obstetrics and Gynecology
Proceedings of the Society of Experimental Biology and Medicine
Quarterly Bulletin, Northwestern University Medical School
Science
Surgical Clinics of Chicago
Surgery Gynecology & Obstetrics (Journal of the American College of Surgeons)
Veterinary Medicine

Bibliography

Newspapers and Magazines

American Urological Association News
The Atlantic
Chicago Daily Tribune
Colliers Magazine
Dallas Times Herald Magazine
Dearborn Independent
Junction City Kansas Union
Kansas City Journal Post
Kansas City Star

New York Times
Newsweek
Pittsburgh Commercial Gazette
Real America Magazine
San Francisco Chronicle
Saturday Review of Literature
Scientific American
Time
Topeka Daily Capital

Other Sources

Correspondence between Alexis Carrel and Serge Voronoff, 1912–13, Special Collections Research Center, Georgetown University Library. Medical Executive Committee Minutes, Chicago Wesley Memorial Hospital, 1946.
Chicago Urological Society Minutes, vol. 1.
Marin County Free Library Oral History Project.

Index

Index

Index